5th edition

comprehensive pharmacy
review practice exams

5th edition

comprehensive pharmacy review practice exams

EDITORS

Alan H. Mutnick, PharmD, RPh, FASHP
Assistant Director, Clinical Pharmacy Services
University of Virginia Health System
Charlottesville, Virginia

Paul F. Souney, MS, RPh
Senior Director Medical Affairs
AstraZeneca LP
Wilmington, Delaware

Larry N. Swanson, PharmD, RPh, FASHP
Professor and Chairman
Department of Pharmacy Practice
Campbell University School of Pharmacy
Buies Creek, North Carolina

Leon Shargel, PhD, RPh
Vice President, Biopharmaceutics
Eon Labs, Inc.
Laurelton, New York
Adjunct Associate Professor
School of Pharmacy
University of Maryland
Baltimore, Maryland

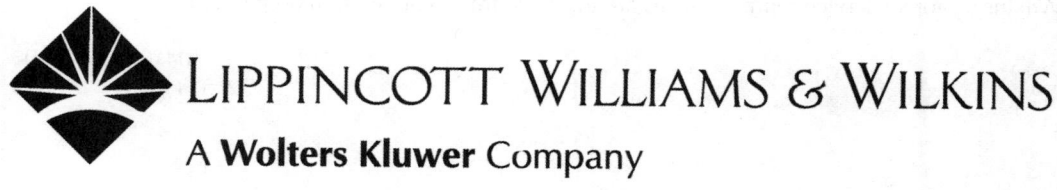

LIPPINCOTT WILLIAMS & WILKINS
A **Wolters Kluwer** Company

Senior Acquisitions Editor: David B. Troy
Senior Managing Editor: Matthew J. Hauber
Marketing Manager: Samantha Smith
Production Editor: Jennifer Ajello
Designer: Risa Clow
Compositor: Graphic World
Printer: Data Reproductions Corp.

351 West Camden Street
Baltimore, MD 21201

530 Walnut Street
Philadelphia, PA 19106

Printed in the United States of America

Library of Congress Cataloging-in-Publication Data

Comprehensive pharmacy review practice exams / editors, Alan H. Mutnick,
Paul F. Souney, Larry N. Swanson ; associate editor, Leon Shargel.—5th ed.
        p. ; cm.
    Companion v. to: Comprehensive pharmacy review. 5th ed.
    ISBN 0-7817-4485-7
    1. Pharmacy—Examinations, questions, etc.
    [DNLM: 1. Pharmacy—Examination Questions.   QV 18.2 C7375 2004]   I.
Mutnick, Alan H.   II. Souney, Paul F.   III. Swanson, Larry N.   IV.
Comprehensive pharmacy review.
    RS97.P49 2003 Suppl.
      615'.4'076—dc22   2003066094

To purchase additional copies of this book, call our customer service department at **(800) 638-3030** or fax orders to **(301) 824-7390**. International customers should call **(301) 714-2324**.

Visit Lippincott Williams & Wilkins on the Internet: http://www.LWW.com. Lippincott Williams & Wilkins customer service representatives are available from 8:30 am to 6:00 pm, EST.

04 05 06 07 08
2 3 4 5 6 7 8 9 10

Contents

Preface

This practice exam booklet is a companion to Comprehensive Pharmacy Review. Whereas Comprehensive Pharmacy Review presents most of the subjects in the pharmacy curriculum in outline form with review questions interspersed, this booklet offers two examinations that are similar in format and coverage to those in the licensing examination required of all pharmacists.

Both patient profile–based and free-standing test items are included in the examinations. The questions are of two general types. In the first type (Example 1), the correct response most accurately completes a statement or answers a question. In the second type (Example 2), three statements are given. The correct answer may include one, two, or all three of these statements; these questions are to be answered according to the direction block that accompanies them.

Example 1 (Multiple-Choice)

Drugs that demonstrate nonlinear pharmacokinetics show which of the following properties?

A. A constant ratio of drug metabolites is formed as the administered dose increases

B. The elimination half-life increases as the administered dose is increased

C. The area under the curve (AUC) increases in direct proportion to an increase in the administered dose

D. Both low and high doses follow first-order elimination kinetics

E. The steady-state drug concentration increases in direct proportion to the dosing rate

Example 2 (Multiple True–False)

Antimuscarinic agents are used in the treatment of Parkinson's disease and in the control of some neuroleptic-induced extrapyramidal disorders. These agents include the following:

I. ipratropium

II. benztropine

III. trihexyphenidyl

A. I only

B. III only

C. I and II

D. II and III

E. I, II, and III

Allow a maximum of four hours for each examination. Answers, with explanations, are given at the end of each exam. Also, several appendices are included at the back of the booklet for reference.

Taking A Test

The necessity of taking a test on the material that has been presented is one of the least attractive aspects of pursuing an education. Examinations are used as a measure of the student's comprehension of the subject matter. Students are required to take many examinations during their learning careers. Little if any time is spent acquainting students with the positive aspects of tests and with systematic and successful methods of approaching them. Students need to view tests as opportunities to display their knowledge and to use them as tools for developing prescriptions for further study and learning.

While preparing for any exam, class and board exams as well as practice exams, it is important that students learn as much as they can about the subject on which they will be tested and discover how much they may not know. Students should study to acquire knowledge, not just to prepare for tests. **For the well-prepared student, the chances of passing far exceed the chances of failing.**

Materials Needed for Test Preparation

In preparing for a test, most students collect far too much study material only to find that they simply do not have time to go through all of it. They are defeated before they begin because they either cannot get through all the material, leaving areas unstudied or they race through the material so quickly that they cannot benefit from the activity.

It is generally more efficient for the student to use materials already at hand; that is, class notes, one good outline to cover and strengthen all areas and to quickly review the whole topic, and one good text as a reference for complex material that requires further explanation.

Also many students attempt to memorize far too much information, rather than learning and understanding basic material and then relying on that learned information to determine the answers to questions at the time of the examination. Relying too heavily on memorized material causes anxiety, and the more anxious students become during a test, the less learned knowledge they are likely to use.

Attitude and Approach

A positive attitude and a realistic approach are essential to successful test taking. If the student's concentration is placed on the negative aspects of tests or on the potential for failure, anxiety increases and performance decreases. A negative attitude generally develops if the student concentrates on "I must pass" rather than "I can pass." "What if I fail?" becomes the major factor motivating the student to **run from failure rather than toward success.** This results from placing too much emphasis on scores. The score received is only one aspect of test performance. Test performance also indicates the student's ability to use differential reasoning.

Test Strategy

In a question with five alternatives, of which one is correct, there are four alternatives that are incorrect. If deductive reasoning is used, the choices can be viewed as having possibilities of being correct. The elimination of wrong choices increases the odds that a student will be able to recognize the correct choice. Even if the correct choice does not become evident, the probability of guessing correctly increases. **Eliminating incorrect choices on a test can result in choosing the correct answer.**

Answering questions based on what is incorrect is difficult for many students since they have had nearly 20 years of experience taking tests with the implied assertion that knowledge can be displayed only by knowing what is correct. It must be remembered, however, that **students can display knowledge by knowing something is wrong, just as they can display it by knowing something is right.**

Preparing for the Examination

1. **Study for yourself.** Although some of the material may seem irrelevant, the more you learn now, the less you will have to learn later. Also, do not let the fear of the test rob you of an important part of your education. If you study to learn, the task is less distasteful than studying solely to pass a test.
2. **Review all areas.** You should not be selective by studying perceived weak areas and ignoring perceived strong areas. Cover all of the material, putting added emphasis on weak areas.
3. **Attempt to understand, not just to memorize, the material.** Ask yourself: To whom does the material apply? When does it apply? Where does it apply? How does it apply? Understanding the connections among these points allows for longer retention and aids in those situations when guessing strategies may be needed.

4. Try to **anticipate questions that might appear on the test.** Ask yourself how you might construct a question on a specific topic.
5. **Give yourself a couple days of rest before the test.** Studying up to the last moment will increase your anxiety and cause potential confusion.

Taking the Examination

1. Be sure to **pace yourself** to use the test time optimally. You should use all of your allotted time; if you finish too early, you may have moved too quickly through the test.
2. **Read each question and all the alternatives carefully** before you begin to make decisions. Remember, the questions contain clues, as do the answer choices.
3. **Read the directions for each question set carefully.** You would be amazed at how many students make mistakes in tests simply because they have not paid close attention to the directions.
4. It is not advisable to leave blanks with the intention of coming back to answer the questions later. If you feel that you must come back to a question, mark the best choice and place a note in the margin. Generally speaking, it is best not to change answers once you have made a decision. Your considered reaction and first response are correct more often than changes made out of frustration or anxiety.
5. **Do not let anxiety destroy your confidence.** If you have prepared conscientiously, you know enough to pass. Use all that you have learned.
6. **Do not try to determine how well you are doing as you proceed.** You will not be able to make an objective assessment, and your anxiety will increase.
7. **Do not become frustrated or angry** about what appear to be bad or difficult questions. You simply do not know the answers; you cannot know everything.

Specific Test-Taking Strategies

Read the entire question carefully, regardless of format. Test questions have multiple parts. Concentrate on picking out the pertinent key words that might help you begin to problem solve. Words such as "always," "all," "never," "mostly," and "primarily," play significant roles. In all types of questions, distractors with terms such as "always" or "never" most often are incorrect. Adjectives and adverbs can completely change the meaning of questions—pay close attention to them. The knowledge and application of grammar often are key to dissecting questions.

Multiple-Choice Questions

Read the question and the choices carefully to become familiar with the data provided. Remember, in multiple-choice questions containing five choices there is one correct answer, and there are four distractors, or incorrect answers. (Distractors are plausible and possibly correct or they would not be called distractors.) Distractors are generally correct for part of the question but not for the entire question. Dissecting the question into parts helps in eliminating distractors.

Many students think that they must always start at option A and make a decision before they move to B, thus forcing decisions they are not ready to make. Your first decisions should be made on those choices you feel the most confident about.

Compare the choices to each part of the question. **To be wrong,** a choice needs to be incorrect for only part of the question. **To be correct,** it must be **totally** correct. If you believe a choice is partially incorrect, tentatively eliminate that choice. Make notes next to the choices regarding tentative decisions. One method is to place a minus sign next to the choices you are certain are incorrect and a plus sign next to those that potentially are correct. Finally, place a zero next to any choice you do not understand or need to come back to for further inspection. Do not feel that you must make final decisions until you have examined all choices carefully.

When you have eliminated as many choices as you can, decide which of those that remain has the highest probability of being correct. Above all, be honest with yourself. If you do not know the answer, eliminate as many choices as possible and choose reasonably.

Multiple True-False Questions

Multiple true-false questions are not as difficult as some students make them. These are the questions for which you must select:

A. if only **I** is correct.
B. if only **III** is correct.
C. if **I** and **II** are correct.
D. if **II** and **III** are correct.
E. if **all** (I, II, and III) are correct.

Remember that the name for this type of question is multiple true-false and then use this concept. Become familiar with each choice and make notes. Then concentrate on the one choice you feel is definitely incorrect. If you can find one incorrect alternative, you can eliminate three choices immediately and be down to a fifty-fifty probability of guessing the correct answer. If choice A is incorrect, so are C and E; if choice B is incorrect so are choices D and E. Therefore, you are down to a fifty-fifty probability of guessing the correct answer.

After eliminating the choices you are sure are incorrect, concentrate on the choice that will make your final decision. For instance, if you discard choice I, you have eliminated alternatives A, C, and E. This leaves B (III) and D (II and III). Concentrate on choice II, and decide if it is true or false. (Take the path of least resistance and concentrate on the smallest possible number of items while making a decision.) Obviously, if none of the choices is found to be incorrect, the answer is E (all).

Guessing

Nothing takes the place of a firm knowledge base, but having little information to work with, you may find it necessary to guess at the correct answer. A few simple rules can help increase your guessing accuracy. Always guess consistently if you have no idea what is correct; that is, after eliminating all that you can, make the choice that agrees with your intuition or choose the option closest to the top of the list that has not been eliminated as a potential answer.

When guessing at questions that present with choices in numeric form, you will often find the choices listed in ascending or descending order. It is generally not wise to guess the first or last alternative, since these are usually extreme values and are most likely incorrect.

Using a Practice Exam to Learn

All too often, students do not take full advantage of practice exams. There is a tendency to complete the exam, score it, look up the correct answer to those questions missed, and then forget the entire thing.

In fact, great educational benefits could be derived if students would spend more time using practice tests as learning tools. As mentioned previously, incorrect choices in test questions are plausible and partially correct or they would not fulfill their purpose as distractors. This means that it is just as beneficial to look up the incorrect choices as the correct choices to discover specifically why they are incorrect. In this way, it is possible to learn better test-taking skills as the subtlety of question construction is uncovered.

In addition, it is advisable to go back and attempt to restructure each question to see if all the choices can be made correct by modifying the question. By doing this, four times as much will be learned. By all means, look up the right answer and explanation. Then, focus on each of the other choices and ask yourself under what conditions they might be correct.

Each exam that follows contains approximately 190 questions and explanations. Every effort has been made to simulate the types of questions and the degree of question difficulty in the board examination. While taking this exam, the student should attempt to create the testing conditions that might be experienced during actual testing situations. Approximately 1 1/2 minutes should be allowed for each question, and the entire test should be finished before it is scored.

Summary

Ideally, examinations are designed to determine how much material students have learned and how that material is used in the successful completion of the examination. Students will be successful if these suggestions are followed:

*   Develop a positive attitude and maintain that attitude.
*   Be realistic in determining the amount of material you attempt to master and in the score you hope to attain.
*   Read the directions for each type of question and the questions themselves closely and follow the directions carefully.
*   Bring differential reasoning to each question in the examination.
*   Guess intelligently and consistently when guessing strategies must be used.
*   Use the test as an opportunity to display your knowledge and as a tool for developing prescriptions for further study and learning.

Board examinations are not easy. They may be almost impossible for those who have unrealistic expectations or for those who allow misinformation concerning the exams to produce anxiety out of proportion to the task at hand. Examinations are manageable if they are approached with a positive attitude and with consistent use of all of the information the student has learned.

Michael J. O'Donnell

INTRODUCTION TO THE NAPLEX™

After graduation from an accredited pharmacy program, the prospective pharmacist must demonstrate the competency to practice pharmacy. The standards of competence for the practice of pharmacy are set by each state board of pharmacy. The NAPLEX™ is the principal instrument used by the state board of pharmacy to assess the knowledge and proficiency necessary for a candidate to practice pharmacy. The National Association of Boards of Pharmacy™ (NABP™) develops examinations that enable boards of pharmacy to assess the competence of candidates seeking licensure to practice pharmacy. Each state board of pharmacy may impose additional examinations. The two major examinations developed by the NABP are:

- The North American Pharmacist Licensure Examination™ (NAPLEX™)
- Multistate Pharmacy Jurisprudence Examination ™ (MPJE™)

Registration information and a description of these computerized examinations may be found on the NABP website: http://www.nabp.org. Prior to submitting registration materials, the pharmacy candidate should contact the board of pharmacy for additional information regarding procedures, deadline dates, and required documentation.

The NAPLEX™ is a computer-adaptive test that measures a candidate's knowledge and ability by assessing the answers before presenting the next test question. If the answer is correct, the computer will select a more difficult question from the test item pool in an appropriate content area; if the answer is incorrect, an easier question will be selected by the computer. The NAPLEX™ score is based on the difficulty level of the questions answered correctly.

NAPLEX™ consists of 185 multiple-choice test questions. Of these, 150 questions are used to calculate the test score. The remaining 35 items serve as pretest questions and do not affect the NAPLEX™ score. Pretest questions are administered to evaluate the item's difficulty level for possible inclusion as a scored question in future exams. These pretest questions are dispersed throughout the exam and cannot be identified by the candidate.

A majority of the questions on the NAPLEX™ are asked in a scenario-based format (i.e., patient profiles with accompanying test questions). To properly analyze and answer the questions presented, the candidate must refer to the information provided in the patient profile. Some questions appear in a stand-alone format and should be answered solely from the information provided in the question.

All NAPLEX™ questions are based on competency statements, that are reviewed and revised periodically. The NAPLEX™ Competency Statements describe the knowledge, judgment, and skills that the candidate is expected to demonstrate as an entry-level pharmacist. A complete description of the NAPLEX™ Competency Statements is published on the NABP website. The NAPLEX™ examines three general areas of competence:

- Management of Drug Therapy to Optimize Patient Outcomes
- Safe and Accurate Preparation and Dispensing of Medications
- Drug Information and Promotion of Public Health

The *NAPLEX™ Candidates' Review Guide* may be obtained from a school or college of pharmacy or from the National Association of Boards of Pharmacy.

Test I

Use the patient profile below to answer questions 1–12.

MEDICATION PROFILE—COMMUNITY

Patient Name: Rachel Sprints
Address: 1923 Crowell
Age: 65   Height: 5'4"
Sex: F   Race: White   Weight: 140 lb
Allergies: Aspirin-related products: anaphylaxis

DIAGNOSIS
Primary   (1)   Status post ST-segment elevated myocardial infarction (STEMI), 9/15
                 (2)
Secondary   (1)   Hypertension
                 (2)   Hypercholesterolemia
                 (3)   Duodenal ulcer

MEDICATION RECORD Prescription and OTC

	Date	R No	Physician	Drug and Strength	Quan	Sig	Refills
(1)	7/20	12233	Johnsie	Niacin 500 mg	30	i tab hs	0
(2)	7/20	12234	Johnsie	Atorvastatin 10 mg	30	i tab hs	6
(3)	7/20	12235	Johnsie	Hydrochlorothiazide 25 mg	30	i tab am	6
(4)	7/20	12236	Johnsie	Aspirin 325 mg	100	i tab am	12
(5)	8/21	14001	Johnsie	Doxazosin 2 mg	30	i tab am	6
(6)	8/21	14002	Johnsie	Ramipril 5 mg	30	i tab am	6
(7)	8/29	15005	Colon	Rabeprazole 20 mg	30	i tab am	0
(8)	9/22	16500	Johnsie	Clopidogrel 75 mg	30	i tab am	6
(9)	9/22	16501	Johnsie	Atenolol 50 mg	30	i tab am	6
(10)	9/22	16502	Johnsie	Nitroglycerin 0.3 mg	100	As directed	6

PHARMACIST NOTES and Other Patient Information

	Date	Comments
(1)	7/20	New patient received from another pharmacy
(2)	7/20	Contacted physician regarding two potential problems with the current prescriptions
(3)	7/20	Physician agreed with both suggestions and acknowledged the oversight.
(4)	7/20	Both medications were discontinued.
(5)	8/21	Contacted physician regarding new prescriptions received, based on findings from the ALLHAT and HOPE studies; however, Dr. Johnsie disagreed with suggestion to delete either of the prescriptions.
(6)	8/21	Patient instructed on proper technique to take blood pressure daily at the same time, prior to taking morning medications, and to make sure prescriptions are refilled promptly each month
(7)	9/22	Updated patient medication profile to reflect current medications, including atorvastatin, hydrochlorothiazide, doxazosin, ramipril, rabeprazole, clopidogrel, atenolol, and nitroglycerin SL.
(8)	9/22	Contacted Dr. Johnsie to reiterate findings from ALLHAT study, and this time he agreed to discontinue the medication.

1. Which medications prompted the pharmacist to call Dr. Johnsie on 7/20 due to potential problems?

   I. Niacin

   II. Atorvastatin

   III. Aspirin

   A. I only

   B. III only

   C. I and II

   D. II and III

   E. I, II, and III

2. Which of the prescriptions written by Dr. Johnsie on 8/21 was the pharmacist hoping to have discontinued, and which study demonstrated its potential negative effects in a hypertensive patient like Ms. Sprints?

   A. Doxazosin and ALLHAT study

   B. Ramipril and ALLHAT study

   C. Doxazosin and HOPE study

   D. Ramipril and HOPE study

   E. Both doxazosin and ramipril in the HOPE study

3. The Joint National Committee-7 guidelines for the treatment of hypertension include "compelling" indications that recommend the use of select drug therapies over standard therapy with a thiazide diuretic. Which of the following choices represent examples of "compelling" indications and their suggested therapy?

   I. Heart failure (diuretics, β-blockers, ACE inhibitors)

   II. Chronic kidney disease (ACE inhibitors, angiotensin II receptor blockers)

   III. Recurrent stroke prevention (diuretics, ACE inhibitors)

   A. I only

   B. III only

   C. I and II

   D. II and III

   E. I, II, and III

4. Which of the following statements would justify the prescription written on 9/22 for atenolol for Ms. Sprints?

   I. Treatment of hypertension in a patient who is post-MI as a compelling indication

   II. Prevention of sudden death in a post-MI patient

   III. Secondary prevention of stroke

   A. I only

   B. III only

   C. I and II

   D. II and III

   E. I, II, and III

5. Which of the following agents, assuming no contraindications for use, was likely to have been given to Ms. Sprints upon arrival to the hospital for the treatment of STEMI, assuming she arrived for treatment within 12 hours of her symptoms?

   I. Recombinant tissue-type plasminogen activator alteplase (t-PA)

   II. Reteplase (r-PA)

   III. Tenecteplase (TNK)

   A. I only

   B. III only

   C. I and II

   D. II and III

   E. I, II, and III

6. After her heart attack, Ms. Sprints presents with a prescription for clopidogrel. What is the indication for clopidogrel in this patient?

   I. Used as an alternative to aspirin due to aspirin allergy

   II. Used in the prevention of acute coronary syndromes

   III. Used in hypertensive patients who have a "compelling" indication

   A. I only

   B. III only

   C. I and II

   D. II and III

   E. I, II, and III

7. Ms. Sprints is receiving rabeprazole for which of the following indications?

    A. Post-MI for prevention of sudden death
    B. Duodenal ulcer
    C. Hypercholesterolemia
    D. Hypertension
    E. None of the above

8. Which of the following patient information items should be addressed when Ms. Sprints receives the nitroglycerin prescription?

    I. The tablet should be dissolved under the tongue if it is difficult to swallow.
    II. The tablets should be placed in an easy-to-open plastic container for future use.
    III. The tablets should be taken for an acute angina attack or prior to an activity that might induce an attack (i.e., strenuous exercise, anxiety).

    A. I only
    B. III only
    C. I and II
    D. II and III
    E. I, II, and III

9. Based on the Joint National Committee-7 guidelines and the antihypertensive therapy being prescribed, which of the following choices best describes Ms. Sprints' blood pressure classification?

    A. Prehypertension
    B. Stage I hypertension
    C. Stage II hypertension
    D. Stage III hypertension
    E. Malignant hypertension

10. Based on Ms. Sprints' patient profile, which of the following medications would be contraindicated in this patient?

    A. Salsalate
    B. Ibuprofen
    C. Celecoxib
    D. Rofecoxib
    E. All of the above

11. Untreated hypertension can result in which of the following types of target-organ damage?

    I. Renal
    II. Cerebral
    III. Retinal

    A. I only
    B. III only
    C. I and II
    D. II and III
    E. I, II, and III

12. Which of the following agents would NOT be considered a first-line antihypertensive agent in an otherwise healthy patient with stage I hypertension?

    A. Amiloride
    B. Chlorthalidone
    C. Chlorothiazide
    D. Indapamide
    E. Methyclothiazide

End of this patient profile; continue with the examination

---

13. Some extended-release theophylline products claim zero-order absorption kinetics. The advantages compared with first-order absorption kinetics include:

    I. More precise plasma concentrations
    II. More complete drug bioavailability
    III. Less plasma drug protein binding

    A. I only
    B. III only
    C. I and II
    D. II and III
    E. I, II, and III

14. H_2-receptor antagonists exert their therapeutic effect by:

    I. Reducing gastric acid secretion
    II. Forming a protective barrier against acid
    III. Decreasing gastrointestinal motility

    A. I only
    B. III only
    C. I and II
    D. II and III
    E. I, II, and III

15. Which statements about insulin resistance are true?

    I. Insulin resistance is the need for more than 200 U/day of insulin.
    II. Insulin resistance can be caused by a high concentration of circulating IgG anti-insulin antibodies.
    III. Insulin resistance can resolve spontaneously.

    A. I only
    B. III only
    C. I and II
    D. II and III
    E. I, II, and III

16. Lanolin is best described as:

    I. A water-in-oil (w/o) emulsion containing approximately 25% water
    II. An emulsion base that acts as an emollient, preventing water loss
    III. A water-soluble base containing propylene glycol or polyethylene glycol, which increases evaporation

    A. I only
    B. III only
    C. I and II
    D. II and III
    E. I, II, and III

17. Which products have been shown to be effective in the treatment of diarrhea?

    I. Donnagel-PG
    II. Kaopectate
    III. Pepto-Bismol

    A. I only
    B. III only
    C. I and II
    D. II and III
    E. I, II, and III

18. Levodopa is preferred to dopamine in the treatment of Parkinson's disease because:

    I. Levodopa crosses the blood–brain barrier; dopamine does not.
    II. Levodopa is a more potent agonist than dopamine at the receptor site in the substantia nigra.
    III. Levodopa is decarboxylated in the gastrointestinal tract, whereas dopamine is not.

    A. I only
    B. III only
    C. I and II
    D. II and III
    E. I, II, and III

19. Which stimulants are approved as OTC agents?

    I. NoDoz
    II. Vivarin
    III. Dexatrim

    A. I only
    B. III only
    C. I and II
    D. II and III
    E. I, II, and III

20. The mechanism of action of salmeterol is that of a:

    A. Sympathomimetic agonist with high β_2 selectivity
    B. Sympathomimetic agonist with high β_1 selectivity
    C. Sympathomimetic antagonist with high β_2 selectivity
    D. Sympathomimetic antagonist with high β_1 selectivity
    E. Leukotriene receptor antagonist

Use the patient profile below to answer questions 21–32.

MEDICATION PROFILE—COMMUNITY

Patient Name: Alan Melvick

Address: 1932 Liberty Lane

Age: 48

Sex: M   Race: White

Height: 5'9"

Weight: 180 lb

Allergies: No known allergies

DIAGNOSIS

Primary   (1)   Heart failure

           (2)

Secondary   (1)   Anemia

           (2)   Anterior myocardial infarction

           (3)

MEDICATION RECORD Prescription and OTC

	Date	℞ No	Physician	Drug and Strength	Quan	Sig	Refills
(1)	6/15	110555	Davis	Prednisone 10 mg	60	i bid	2
(2)	8/10	111002	Davis	Ferrous sulfate 325 mg	100	i tid	6
(3)	8/10	111003	Zielger	Lanoxin 0.25 mg	30	i q AM	6
(4)	8/10	111004	Ziegler	Lasix 40 mg	30	i q AM	3
(5)	8/10	111005	Ziegler	Slow-K 600 mg	90	i tid	3
(6)	9/10	113001	Ziegler	Vasotec 5 mg	30	i qd	3
(7)	9/10	113002	Ziegler	Hydrochlorothiazide 50 mg	30	i bid	3
(8)	9/10	113002	Ziegler	Isordil 40 mg	120	i qid	3
(9)	9/10	113003	Ziegler	Hydralazine 50 mg	60	i bid	3
(10)	12/1	200001	Ziegler	Coreg 3.125 mg	30	i bid	0
(11)	12/1	200002	Ziegler	Altace 2.5 mg	30	i q AM	0
(12)	12/15	200604	Ziegler	Coreg 6.25 mg	30	i bid	0
(13)	1/2	201003	Ziegler	Altace 5.0 mg	30	i q AM	3
(14)	1/2	201004	Ziegler	Coreg 12.5 mg	60	i bid	0
(15)	1/16	203010	Abrams	Micro K 20 mEq	30	i q AM	6

PHARMACIST NOTES and Other Patient Information

	Date	Comments
(1)	9/10	Patient presents with new prescriptions and told pharmacist that Dr. Ziegler wanted him to stop taking the Lanoxin.
(2)	9/10	Pharmacist contacted Dr. Ziegler with questions about several of the prescriptions in patient profile as well as new prescriptions presented to pharmacy.
(3)	9/10	D/C Lasix
(4)	9/10	D/C Lanoxin
(5)	9/10	D/C Slow-K 600
	12/1	D/C Isordil 40 mg, hydralazine 50 mg, and Vasotec 5 mg
(6)	12/15	Pharmacist contacted Dr. Ziegler regarding Coreg prescription initially filled on 12/1, and received requested verbal prescription.
(7)	1/2	Contacted Dr. Ziegler regarding indication for new Altace prescription
(8)	1/16	Pharmacist contacted Dr. Abrams regarding recently prescribed potassium supplement.

21. Based on the medication profile presented on 8/10, which choices describe potential etiologies for Mr. Melvick's heart failure?

    I. Low-output failure caused by myocardial infarction
    II. Low-output failure caused by prednisone
    III. High-output failure caused by anemia

    A. I only
    B. III only
    C. I and II
    D. II and III
    E. I, II, and III

22. Which choices describe the interaction that should have taken place when Mr. Melvick was having his prescriptions filled on 9/10?

    I. No significant interaction is needed with the new prescriptions.
    II. The pharmacist should advise Dr. Ziegler of the interaction between isosorbide dinitrate and hydralazine.
    III. The pharmacist should call Dr. Ziegler regarding the combination of Slow-K and Vasotec.

    A. I only
    B. III only
    C. I and II
    D. II and III
    E. I, II, and III

23. Why did the pharmacist contact Dr. Ziegler on 12/15 regarding the Coreg prescription?

    I. Coreg is a member of the angiotensin-2 receptor blockers, which currently are not indicated in the treatment of heart failure.
    II. Coreg is a β-adrenergic blocker, and in the treatment of heart failure the dose must be titrated up to the optimal dose.
    III. β-adrenergic blockers should not be abruptly discontinued in cardiac patients.

    A. I only
    B. III only
    C. I and II
    D. II and III
    E. I, II, and III

24. Which group of symptoms is most often associated with a patient who has signs of left-sided heart failure?

    A. Shortness of breath, rales, paroxysmal nocturnal dyspnea
    B. Jugular venous distention, hepatojugular reflux, pedal edema, shortness of breath
    C. Hepatojugular reflux, jugular venous distention, pedal edema, abdominal distention
    D. Paroxysmal nocturnal dyspnea, pedal edema, jugular venous distention, hepatojugular reflux
    E. Fatigue, abdominal distention, hepatomegaly, rales

25. What is the therapeutic indication for Altace that prompted the pharmacist's call to Dr. Ziegler on 1/2?

    A. Hypertension
    B. Renal dysfunction
    C. Heart failure
    D. Cardiovascular risk reduction
    E. Peripheral vascular disease

26. How many milligrams of elemental iron does Mr. Melvick receive with his daily dose of ferrous sulfate?

    A. 117 mg
    B. 195 mg
    C. 150 mg
    D. 322 mg
    E. 975 mg

27. Which action best describes how the drug Lasix would affect Mr. Melvick?

    I. Reduction of excess sodium and water in the patient
    II. Direct pulmonary dilation
    III. Increased preload through cytokine release

    A. I only
    B. III only
    C. I and II
    D. II and III
    E. I, II, and III

28. Which pharmacologic mechanisms relate primarily to the use of Vasotec in this patient?

    I. Angiotensin-converting enzyme inhibitors indirectly reduce preload by decreasing aldosterone secretion.
    II. Angiotensin-converting enzyme inhibitors reduce afterload by decreasing angiotensin II production.
    III. Angiotensin-converting enzyme inhibitors decrease levels of bradykinin.

    A. I only
    B. III only
    C. I and II
    D. II and III
    E. I, II, and III

29. What is the major difference between Lanoxin tablets and Lanoxicaps capsules?

    I. The digoxin contained in Lanoxicaps capsules is more potent than the digoxin contained in Lanoxin tablets.
    II. The digoxin contained in Lanoxicaps capsules is more completely absorbed than is the digoxin in Lanoxin tablets.
    III. Digoxin absorption from Lanoxicaps capsules is less variable than is digoxin absorption from Lanoxin tablets.

    A. I only
    B. III only
    C. I and II only
    D. II and III only
    E. I, II, and III

30. Which drug used in the treatment of heart failure has been associated with systemic lupus erythematosus?

    A. Apresoline
    B. Lanoxin
    C. Vasotec
    D. Lasix
    E. Isordil

31. Which of the following drugs represent the class of drugs recently given a Class III recommendation that stated, "that conditions for which there is evidence and/or general agreement that a procedure/therapy is not useful/effective and in some cases may be harmful" in the treatment of heart failure?

    I. Inocor
    II. Dobutrex
    III. Dopamine

    A. I only
    B. III only
    C. I and II
    D. II and III
    E. I, II, and III

32. Which statements best represent the actions that a pharmacist should take if presented with a prescription for Motrin for Mr. Melvick?

    I. Contact the physician regarding the history of anemia in the patient.
    II. Contact the physician regarding the allergy to aspirin reported on the medication profile for the patient.
    III. Fill the prescription, and counsel the patient on the correct method for taking the ibuprofen with meals.

    A. I only
    B. III only
    C. I and II
    D. II and III
    E. I, II, and III

End of this patient profile; continue with the examination

33. Which of the following statements does NOT accurately describe the current role that β-adrenergic blockers play in the treatment of heart failure?

    A. β-adrenergic blockers have been shown to decrease the risk of death or hospitalization as well as improve the clinical status of heart failure patients.

    B. Current guidelines recommend the use of β-adrenergic blockers in all patients with stable heart failure due to left ventricular dysfunction unless they have a contraindication to their use or are unable to tolerate their effects due to hypotension, bradycardia, bronchospasm, and the like.

    C. β-adrenergic blockers are generally used in conjunction with diuretics and angiotensin-converting enzyme (ACE) inhibitors.

    D. Side effects to β-adrenergic blockers may occur during the early days of therapy but do not generally prevent their long-term use, and progression of the disease may be reduced.

    E. β-adrenergic blockers are contraindicated in the treatment of heart failure due to their strong negative inotropic effects, which further reduce cardiac output.

34. The use of atropine sulfate in the treatment of sinus bradycardia centers around its anticholinergic activity. What hemodynamic response should be monitored for when the drug is administered?

    A. Initial doses may cause constipation.
    B. High doses will cause pupillary constriction.
    C. Initial doses may exacerbate the bradycardia.
    D. High doses will cause diarrhea.
    E. Initial doses will cause extreme sweating.

35. Which cardiac drugs are available in extended-release dosage forms?

    I. Quinaglute
    II. Coreg
    III. Plendil

    A. I only
    B. III only
    C. I and II
    D. II and III
    E. I, II, and III

36. Which agents would be alternate therapy in an intensive care unit patient nonresponsive to dopamine or dobutamine?

    A. Blocadren
    B. Calan
    C. Norpace
    D. Inocor
    E. Tenormin

37. Which agent works by irreversibly blocking the proton pump of parietal cells, thereby inhibiting basal gastric acid secretion?

    A. Tagamet
    B. Carafate
    C. Sandostatin
    D. Prevacid
    E. Pepcid

38. The serum creatinine level, along with the age, weight, and gender of the patient, may be used to estimate creatinine clearance. Creatinine clearance is a measurement of:

    A. Glomerular filtration rate (GFR)
    B. Active tubular secretion
    C. Muscle metabolism
    D. Hepatic function
    E. Effective renal plasma flow

39. Which agents may induce an acute attack of gout?

    I. Low-dose aspirin
    II. Nicotinic acid
    III. Cytotoxic drugs

    A. I only
    B. III only
    C. I and II
    D. II and III
    E. I, II, and III

40. When used as a topical decongestant, oxymetazoline:

    I. Is recommended for administration every 12 hours
    II. Has limited use, generally 3 days or less
    III. Acts as a direct-acting parasympatho-mimetic agent

    A. I only
    B. III only
    C. I and II
    D. II and III
    E. I, II, and III

41. Iron in the form of ferrous salts is often used in the treatment of anemia. Other names for ferrous gluconate include:

    I. Fergon
    II. Feosol
    III. Femiron

    A. I only
    B. III only
    C. I and II
    D. II and III
    E. I, II, and III

Use the patient profile below to answer questions 42–57.

MEDICATION PROFILE—COMMUNITY

Patient Name: ___Chuck Johnson___

Address: ___245 Conway St.___

Age: ___66___

Sex: ___M___   Race: ___White___   Height: ___5'9"___

                                                            Weight: ___172 lb___

Allergies: ___No known allergies___

DIAGNOSIS

Primary	(1)	Diabetes mellitus
	(2)	Osteoarthritis
	(3)	Insomnia
Secondary	(1)	Hx of peptic ulcer disease
	(2)	

MEDICATION RECORD Prescription and OTC

	Date	Rx No	Physician	Drug and Strength	Quan	Sig	Refills
(1)	1/12			Tylenol 500 mg	100	1-2 prn	OTC
(2)	1/30			Nytol Quickgels 50 mg	24	1 hs prn	OTC
(3)	2/10	20101	Jones	Sonata 5 mg	20	1 hs prn	1
(4)	3/6	21134	Jones	Glyburide 5 mg	30	1 q am	3
(5)	6/19	22453	Jones	Metformin 500 mg	60	1 bid	3
(6)	6/19		Jones	Tylenol 500 mg	100	2 q6h max.	OTC
(7)	7/12			Robitussin Cold Multisymptom Cold & Flu Caplets	12	1 q4h prn	OTC
(8)	8/30	23100	Jones	Tramadol 50 mg	40	1/2 tab to start	2
(9)	9/7	25398	Jones	Acarbose 25 mg	90	1 tid	3

PHARMACIST NOTES and Other Patient Information

	Date	Comments
(1)	1/12	Patient complains of some pain in his right knee; he indicates that there is no redness or swelling; recommended Tylenol to treat.
(2)	1/30	Patient complains of insomnia; recommended Nytol 50 mg.
(3)	3/6	Patient has oral glucose tolerance test.
(4)	7/12	Patient reports symptoms of a common cold.
(5)	9/7	Patient reports SMBG high after meals.

42. There are four clinical classes of diabetes mellitus. Which of the following BEST identifies three of these four clinical classes?

    A. Type 1, Type 2, hyperglycemia
    B. Prediabetes, hyperglycemic hyperosmolar nonketotic syndrome (HHNK), Type 3
    C. Gestational diabetes mellitus, Type 1, Type 2
    D. Cushing's syndrome, diabetic ketoacidosis, thiazide diuretic diabetes
    E. Prediabetes, gestational diabetes mellitus, ketonemia

43 Diagnostic criteria used to make the diagnosis of diabetes mellitus in this patient would include:

    I. A fasting plasma glucose level of greater than or equal to 126 mg/dl
    II. A random plasma glucose level greater than or equal to 200 mg/dl with the classic symptoms of diabetes of polydipsia, polyuria, and polyphagia, and weight loss
    III. A 2-hour plasma glucose level of 140 mg/dl during an oral glucose tolerance test using 75 g anhydrous glucose dissolved in water

    A. I only
    B. III only
    C. I and II
    D. II and III
    E. I, II, and III

44. Mr. Johnson indicates to you that his physician said something about a "hemoglobin-type test to check how my blood sugar was doing." Which of the following applies to hemoglobin A1C in diabetes?

    I. A value of <7% (based on 6% as the upper limit of normal) would be a desired therapeutic endpoint.
    II. Another name for this is the glycosylated hemoglobin test.
    III. This reflects the average blood glucose level over the preceding 2 to 3 months.

    A. I only
    B. III only
    C. I and II
    D. II and III
    E. I, II, and III

45. Glyburide is an example of:

    I. An oral insulin secretagogue
    II. An oral hypoglycemic agent
    III. A sulfonylurea

    A. I only
    B. III only
    C. I and II
    D. II and III
    E. I, II, and III

46. Glyburide is also known as:

    I. Diabeta
    II. Micronase
    III. Glucotrol

    A. I only
    B. III only
    C. I and II
    D. II and III
    E. I, II, and III

47. Which of the following information applies to the prescription for metformin given to Mr. Johnson?

    I. It can be used in combination with glyburide.
    II. It is classified as an insulin sensitizer.
    III. It is contraindicated in situations with the potential for increased risk of lactic acidosis.

    A. I only
    B. III only
    C. I and II
    D. II and III
    E. I, II, and III

48. Why would acarbose be added to the other agents used to treat this patient?

    I. Because Mr. Johnson probably has significant postprandial hyperglycemia
    II. Because this agent helps to lower the baseline blood glucose level
    III. Because this agent has a similar mechanism of action as metformin

    A. I only
    B. III only
    C. I and II
    D. II and III
    E. I, II, and III

49. Mr. Johnson is not excited about sticking his finger to check his blood glucose and asks you about testing his urine sugar levels like his aunt used to do. You should tell him:

    I. "Urine glucose testing is no longer recommended since it only provides past (retrospective) blood glucose information and does not reflect current blood glucose."
    II. "Because you have Type 2 diabetes, it is OK to just check your urine sugar."
    III. "With your situation, you really only need to check for ketones in the urine."

    A. I only
    B. III only
    C. I and II
    D. II and III
    E. I, II, and III

50. Mr. Johnson apparently has osteoarthritis in his right knee. Which of the following is/are characteristic of osteoarthritis?

    I. It was formerly known as degenerative joint disease.
    II. It is the most common form of arthritis.
    III. It has a significant inflammatory component.

    A. I only
    B. III only
    C. I and II
    D. II and III
    E. I, II, and III

51. Mr. Johnson requested something to help him with his sleep problem. Which of the following applies to Mr. Johnson and his use of Nytol Quickgels?

    I. This product contains diphenhydramine as the active ingredient.
    II. This product should be used cautiously in the elderly because of potential adverse central anticholinergic effects.
    III. As an elderly man, Mr. Johnson may have prostate enlargement and this agent may produce polyuria, which could confuse the interpretation of his diabetes symptoms.

    A. I only
    B. III only
    C. I and II
    D. II and III
    E. I, II, and III

52. Mr. Johnson was prescribed Sonata for his insomnia. Which of the following applies to this agent?

    I. It has a long half-life and is therefore useful for patients who have difficulty staying asleep.
    II. It would be particularly useful for patients having difficulty falling asleep.
    III. He has received the lower strength of this agent, which is probably good since he is an elderly gentleman.

    A. I only
    B. III only
    C. I and II
    D. II and III
    E. I, II, and III

53. Which of the following agents is considered the first-line therapy for osteoarthritis?

    A. Ibuprofen
    B. Acetaminophen
    C. Naproxen
    D. Codeine
    E. Celecoxib

54. Is the dose selected for this patient an appropriate one to treat the osteoarthritis?

    A. Yes
    B. No

55. Which of the following applies to tramadol?

    I. Mr. Johnson was likely begun on this agent instead of an NSAID because of his history of peptic ulcer disease.
    II. Tramadol is considered a good choice when the patient cannot take an NSAID.
    III. Although not considered an opioid, its side effects are similar.

    A. I only
    B. III only
    C. I and II
    D. II and III
    E. I, II, and III

56. Giving Robitussin Cold Multisymptom Cold & Flu Caplets to Mr. Johnson to treat his common cold symptoms would not be recommended because:

    I. The oral decongestant in this product may cause an elevation in his blood sugar.

    II. It is "shotgun" therapy; one usually should treat specific symptoms with single-agent products.

    III. It contains acetaminophen, which may push Mr. Johnson into a toxic dose.

    A. I only
    B. III only
    C. I and II
    D. II and III
    E. I, II, and III

57. Which of Mr. Johnson's diabetes medications is/are prone to primary and secondary failure?

    I. Glyburide
    II. Metformin
    III. Acarbose

    A. I only
    B. III only
    C. I and II
    D. II and III
    E. I, II, and III

End of this patient profile; continue with the examination

---

58. Jean, a regular customer in your pharmacy, shows you her newborn baby's head and asks you to recommend treatment. Upon examining the baby, you notice that he has an accumulation of skin scales on the scalp. You tell her that the baby has cradle cap and recommend that she treat the baby by:

    A. Washing the baby's head with coal tar solution daily for 2 weeks
    B. Washing his head with an antifungal shampoo (Nizoral AD)
    C. Applying topical antibiotics such as Neosporin daily until resolved
    D. Massaging the scalp with baby oil followed by washing his head with a mild shampoo, such as Johnson & Johnson's baby shampoo
    E. Applying a moisturizer to the scalp daily until resolved

59. Sunscreens should generally not be used in children younger than 6 months because:

    A. They commonly cause a severe rash in this age group.
    B. They produce too much sweat, which can dilute the sunscreen.
    C. The metabolic and excretory systems of infants are not fully developed.
    D. Overexposure to the sun can interfere with vitamin D production.
    E. Infants have a lot of dermal melanin, which causes them to burn more easily.

60. Common warts are treated with which acid?

    A. Glycolic acid
    B. Salicylic acid
    C. Lactic acid
    D. Muriatic acid
    E. Galactic acid

61. Which virus below is responsible for common warts?

    A. Herpes simplex virus
    B. Epstein-Barr virus
    C. Coronavirus
    D. HIV
    E. Human papillomavirus

62. Pyrantel pamoate is indicated for the treatment of pinworms. Besides treatment with this agent, other precautions must be used when a child has pinworms. Related to the treatment of this condition, all the following statements are correct EXCEPT:

    A. Pyrantel pamoate paralyzes the worms through depolarization of muscle.
    B. All household members should be treated.
    C. All bedrooms should be thoroughly swept with a broom.
    D. Clothes and linens should be washed in hot water.
    E. Children should take showers rather than baths.

Use the patient profile below to answer questions 63–71.

PATIENT RECORD—INSTITUTION/NURSING HOME

Patient Name: Salvatore Torres
Address: 1426 8th Street
Age: 55   Height: 5"10'
Sex: M   Race: White   Weight: 170 lb
Allergies: Sulfa drug-induced Stevens-Johnson syndrome

DIAGNOSIS

Primary   (1)   Hypertension
              (2)
Secondary   (1)   Drug-induced erythema multiforme
              (2)   Status post acute coronary syndrome
              (3)   Asthma

LAB/DIAGNOSTIC TESTS

	Date	Test		Date	Test
(1)	11/3	WBC 5500/mm^3	(7)		
(2)	11/3	BUN 15 mg/dl	(8)		
(3)	11/3	Creatinine 1.0 mg/dl	(9)		
(4)	11/3	Blood pressure 170/100	(10)		
(5)	11/3	Electrolytes are within normal limits	(11)		
(6)	11/5	Total cholesterol 250, elevated LDL	(12)		

MEDICATION ORDERS Including Parenteral Solutions

	Date	Comments	Route	Sig
(1)	11/3	Atenolol 50 mg	po	i bid
(2)	11/3	Hydrochlorothiazide (HCTZ) 50 mg	po	i q AM
(3)	11/3	Nitroglycerin 1/150	sl	prn
(4)	11/3	Spironolactone 50 mg	po	i bid
(5)	11/3	Theo-Dur 200 mg	po	i tid
(6)	11/5	Irbesartan 150 mg	po	i qd
(7)	11/5	Simvastatin 40 mg	po	i hs
(8)	11/5	Nitroprusside infusion	IV	i mcg/kg/min titrated
(9)	11/5	Morphine sulfate	IM	prn chest pain

ADDITIONAL ORDERS

	Date	Comments
(1)		
(2)		

DIETARY CONSIDERATIONS Enteral and Parentral

	Date	Comments
(1)	11/3	Low-fat American Heart Association diet
(2)	11/3	Limit sodium intake to no additional salt with meals

PHARMACIST NOTES and Other Patient Information

	Date	Comments
(1)	11/3	D/C HCTZ and replace with spironolactone
(2)	11/5	Blood pressure not responding to initial therapy; begin nitroprusside infusion
(3)	11/5	Begin lipid lowering therapy
(4)	11/5	Schedule for coronary catheterization in the morning

63. Which of the following selections represents the medication of choice for the initial therapy of Stage I hypertension in an otherwise healthy individual with no compelling indications?

    A. Hydrochlorothiazide
    B. Spironolactone
    C. Doxazosin
    D. Hydralazine
    E. Clonidine

64. The decision to discontinue hydrochlorothiazide therapy and begin spironolactone therapy was due to which of the following reasons?

    I. Inappropriate therapeutic effect by thiazide diuretics in hypertensive patients
    II. Lack of proven benefit in reducing mortality rates with diuretics in treating hypertension
    III. Patient's documented allergy to sulfa drug-induced Stevens-Johnson syndrome

    A. I only
    B. III only
    C. I and II
    D. II and III
    E. I, II, and III

65. Which of the following is NOT a major determinant of myocardial oxygen demand?

    A. Heart rate
    B. Myocardial contractility
    C. Coronary blood flow
    D. Left ventricular volume
    E. Myocardial wall tension

66. Which of the following symptoms represents an example of an acute coronary syndrome?

    I. Unstable angina
    II. STEMI
    III. NSTEMI

    A. I only
    B. III only
    C. I and II
    D. II and III
    E. I, II, and III

67. Theophylline serum levels are increased by all of the following EXCEPT:

    A. Pneumonia
    B. Ciprofloxacin
    C. Heart failure
    D. Smoking
    E. Cor pulmonale

68. Due to the fact that Mr. Torres has a secondary diagnosis of asthma, which of the following medications might need to be avoided due to a potential contraindication in asthmatic patients?

    I. Spironolactone
    II. Irbesartan
    III. Atenolol

    A. I only
    B. III only
    C. I and II
    D. II and III
    E. I, II, and III

69. Which of the following agents slows electrical conduction through the atrioventricular node of the heart and has been used for treating hypertension and tachyarrhythmias, as well as angina pectoris?

    A. Amlodipine
    B. Nifedipine
    C. Felodipine
    D. Verapamil
    E. Isradipine

70. Which of the following currently available agents has been shown to be effective in reducing low-density lipoprotein (LDL) cholesterol levels with a resultant reduction in the mortality rate from coronary artery disease in patients with hypercholesterolemia?

    I. Cerivastatin
    II. Pravastatin
    III. Simvastatin

    A. I only
    B. III only
    C. I and II
    D. II and III
    E. I, II, and III

71. Olmesartan represents which of the following drug classes currently available for the treatment of hypertension?

    I. Centrally acting α-adrenergic agonists

    II. Cardiospecific β-adrenergic receptor blocking agents

    III. Angiotensin II type I receptor antagonists

    A. I only
    B. III only
    C. I and II
    D. II and III
    E. I, II, and III

Use the patient profile below to answer questions 72–82.

PATIENT RECORD—INSTITUTION/NURSING HOME

Patient Name: Horace Crenshaw
Address: 3549 Lakeside Dr
Age: 71   Height: 5'2"
Sex: M   Race: White   Weight: 125 lb
Allergies: No known allergies

DIAGNOSIS

Primary	(1)	2-year history Parkinson's disease
	(2)	
Secondary	(1)	Narrow-angle glaucoma
	(2)	30-year history of hypertension
	(3)	Gastroesophageal reflux disease

LAB/DIAGNOSTIC TESTS

	Date	Test		Date	Test
(1)	6/20	Na 135; K 3.6; Cl 95; CO_2 24; BUN 18; Cr 1.3	(4)		
(2)	6/20	Occult blood in stool, negative	(5)		
(3)	6/20	Blood pressure 150/85	(6)		

MEDICATION ORDERS Including Parenteral Solutions

	Date	Comments	Route	Sig
(1)	6/20	Acetazolamide SR 500 mg	po	i qd
(2)	6/20	Levodopa/Carbidopa 25/250	po	i tid
(3)	6/20	Pilocarpine 4%	ophthalmic	gtt i ou q 6 h
(4)	6/20	Reserpine 0.25 mg	po	i qd
(5)	6/20	Diltiazem 30 mg	po	i tid
(6)	6/20	Vitamin B complex w/vitamin C	po	i qd
(7)	7/20	Entacapone Tablets	po	200 mg daily
(8)	12/20	Tolcapone	po	100 mg tid

ADDITIONAL ORDERS

	Date	Comments
(1)	12/20	Baseline LFTs
(2)		

DIETARY CONSIDERATIONS Enteral and Parentral

	Date	Comments
(1)		
(2)		

PHARMACIST NOTES and Other Patient Information

	Date	Comments
(1)	12/20	D/C Entacapone tablets
(2)		

72. Mr. Crenshaw has Parkinson's disease, which is a slowly progressive, degenerative, neurologic disease characterized by tremor, rigidity, bradykinesia, and postural instability. Although this disease is primarily idiopathic in etiology, secondary parkinsonism may be caused by:

    I. Dopamine antagonists (e.g., phenothiazines, butyrophenones)
    II. Poisoning by chemicals (e.g., carbon monoxide poisoning, manganese, or mercury)
    III. Infectious diseases (e.g., viral encephalitis, syphilis)

    A. I only
    B. III only
    C. I and II
    D. II and III
    E. I, II, and III

73. Mr. Crenshaw's physician wants to initiate antihistamine therapy to treat the mild tremor that was the initial parkinsonian symptom experienced. Which antihistamines would be suitable?

    I. Amantadine
    II. Trihexyphenidyl
    III. Diphenhydramine

    A. I only
    B. III only
    C. I and II
    D. II and III
    E. I, II, and III

74. The physician selects biperiden rather than the antihistamine to treat Mr. Crenshaw's initial symptoms. The usual daily dosage range for biperiden is:

    A. 1.0–6.0 mg/day
    B. 1.5–4.5 mg/day
    C. 2.0–8.0 mg/day
    D. 300–600 mg/day
    E. 200–1600 mg/day

75. Upon the monthly medical record review by the local pharmacist, a notation is made to follow up with the medical staff on the recent order written for entacapone on 7/20. What place does entacapone have in the treatment of Parkinson's disease?

    I. Entacapone is indicated as an adjunct to levodopa/carbidopa to treat patients with end-of-dose "wearing off" symptoms.
    II. Entacapone is an enhancer of the bioavailability of levodopa.
    III. Entacapone is a precursor to dopamine indicated in the treatment of refractory Parkinson's.

    A. I only
    B. III only
    C. I and II
    D. II and III
    E. I, II, and III

76. The physician has some concerns regarding the use of anticholinergics in Mr. Crenshaw. Of what precautions in their use should the pharmacist inform the physician?

    A. Complications of narrow-angle glaucoma
    B. Consequences of fluid loss from diarrhea
    C. Urinary incontinence
    D. Excessive salivation
    E. Excessive central nervous system excitation

77. Typical side effects associated with the use of levodopa include:

    I. Gastrointestinal effects, including anorexia, nausea and vomiting, and abdominal distress
    II. Cardiovascular effects, including postural hypotension and tachycardia
    III. Musculoskeletal effects, including dystonia or choreiform muscle movements

    A. I only
    B. III only
    C. I and II
    D. II and III
    E. I, II, and III

78. When using anticholinergic therapy for the treatment of this patient's parkinsonian tremor, which therapeutic considerations are applicable?

    I. Anticholinergic agents are best used in combination to maximize benefits.
    II. Trihexyphenidyl is generally the most effective anticholinergic agent for the treatment of parkinsonian tremor.
    III. Changing to another anticholinergic agent may not prove helpful if the therapeutic effect of the first agent is unsatisfactory, but changing to a different drug class may be beneficial.

    A. I only
    B. III only
    C. I and II
    D. II and III
    E. I, II, and III

79. Based on the patient's medical history before admission, the physician concludes that anticholinergic or antihistamine therapy is insufficient. Dopaminergic therapy could be instituted in the form of:

    A. Chlorphenoxamine
    B. Biperiden
    C. Mesoridazine
    D. Pergolide
    E. Perphenazine

80. Levodopa is metabolized to dopamine by dopa-decarboxylase both centrally and peripherally. This metabolism could be a potential complication for this patient because of:

    A. Concomitant vitamin B complex therapy
    B. Elevated serum creatinine level
    C. Concomitant diltiazem therapy
    D. Concomitant vitamin C therapy
    E. Elevated blood pressure

81. In choosing dopaminergic therapy for this patient, the physician considers giving the combination of carbidopa and levodopa therapy. This combination serves to:

    I. Inhibit peripheral decarboxylation of levodopa to dopamine
    II. Increase the required dose of levodopa by approximately 25%
    III. Decrease the amount of levodopa available for transport to the brain

    A. I only
    B. III only
    C. I and II
    D. II and III
    E. I, II, and III

82. An adjunctive therapeutic regimen for Mr. Crenshaw, relative to his previous "on-off" history, would be:

    A. Monthly interruption of levodopa therapy (drug holiday) on either an inpatient or an outpatient basis
    B. Addition of bromocriptine in a dosage range of 2.5 to 40 mg/day
    C. Addition of amantadine in a dose tailored to the level of renal function
    D. Addition of a monoamine oxidase inhibitor
    E. Addition of haloperidol in a dosage range of 2.5 to 15 mg/day

---

End of this patient profile; continue with the examination

Treatment	C_{max} (mcg/ml)	AUC (0–24 hr) (mcg × hr/ml)	T_{max} (hr)
Fasting	95 ± 10	450 ± 115	1.5 ± 1.1
With antacid	106 ± 18	498 ± 123	1.0 ± 1.2
With high-fat breakfast	75 ± 11*	423 ± 110	2.4 ± 1.3*

Results are expressed as the mean ± SD.
*Compared with fasting, $p \le 0.05$.

83. The effects of food and antacid on the bioavailability of a new antihypertensive agent were studied in 24 men, using a three-way crossover design. The results of this study are summarized in the table above. Compared with fasting, what results did the study show?

  I. The high-fat breakfast had no significant effect on the bioavailability of the drug.
  II. The antacid significantly increased the extent of systemic drug absorption.
  III. The high-fat breakfast treatment decreased the rate of systemic drug absorption.

  A. I only
  B. III only
  C. I and II
  D. II and III
  E. I, II, and III

84. An example of a nitrogen mustard is:

  A. Chlorambucil
  B. Busulfan
  C. Melphalan
  D. Mechlorethamine
  E. Doxorubicin

85. A controlled-release dosage form where the mechanism for drug release is due to an osmotically active drug core is known as:

  A. Dospan
  B. OROS
  C. TDDS
  D. Pennkinetic
  E. HBS

86. All of the following are quinolone antimicrobials EXCEPT:

  A. Moxifloxacin
  B. Levofloxacin
  C. Clarithromycin
  D. Ciprofloxacin
  E. Gatifloxacin

87. Which immunosuppressive agents are used after kidney transplantation?

  I. Azathioprine
  II. Basiliximab
  III. Cyclosporine

  A. I only
  B. III only
  C. I and II
  D. II and III
  E. I, II, and III

PATIENT RECORD—INSTITUTION/NURSING HOME

Patient Name: Sandra Cunningham
Address: 3345 Washington Street
Age: 72   Height: 5'4"
Sex: F   Race: White   Weight: 110 lb
Allergies: Quinidine, tinnitus, blurred vision, headache, nausea; Diuril: rash

DIAGNOSIS

Primary   (1) Acute myocardial infarction
            (2)
Secondary   (1) Hypertension
            (2) Hypothyroidism

LAB/DIAGNOSTIC TESTS

	Date	Test		Date	Test
(1)	3/20	EKG stat and at completion of t-PA therapy; baseline ST segment increase in II, III, and aVF	(7)	3/20	INR, aPTT stat, and then at 6 and 12 hours after completion of t-PA; aPTT at baseline 30 seconds, 6 hours > 120; INR at baseline 1
(2)	3/20	CBC: WBC count 12,000			
(3)	3/20	Platelet count 240,000	(8)	3/20	Urinalysis stat, and then at 6 hours; baseline WNL
(4)	3/20	Chem 20			
(5)	3/20	Cardiac enzymes stat, at 6 and 12 hours; baseline 1500 IU, peak 2566 IU	(9)	3/22	T_4, 1.8 µg/dl
			(10)	3/22	T_3 resin uptake 38%
(6)	3/20	CK-MB fraction stat, at 6 and 12 hours; baseline 32 IU, peak 166 IU	(11)		
			(12)		

MEDICATION ORDERS Including Parenteral Solutions

	Date	Comments	Route	Sig
(1)	3/20	Chewable ASA 80 mg	po	× 2 ASAP
(2)	3/20	Heparin 5000 U	IV	as one time only bolus
(3)	3/20	Heparin 1000 U	IV	qh as continuous infusion
(4)	3/20	t-PA 15 mg	IVP	followed by 37.50 mg continuous IV infusion over 30 minutes, followed by 25 mg over 60 minutes
5)	3/20	Atenolol 5 mg	IV	over 5 minutes, repeated in 10 minutes
(6)	3/20	Atenolol 50 mg	po	10 minutes after last IV dose
(7)	3/20	Captopril 25 mg	po	i tid
(8)	3/20	Docusate 50-mg capsules	po	ii hs
(9)	3/20	Reduce heparin infusion to 800 U	IV	qh
(10)	3/20	Levothyroxine 0.3 mg	po	q AM
(11)	3/20	Continue amiodarone as at home 200 mg	po	ii qd
(12)	3/23	Captopril 6.25 mg	po	1 then 12.5 mg tid thereafter

DIETARY CONSIDERATIONS Enteral and Parenteral

	Date	Comments
(1)	3/20	Low-salt, low-fat diet
(2)	3/22	Extra fiber

PHARMACIST NOTES and Other Patient Information

	Date	Comments
(1)	3/20	BP 150/100, pulse 120, respirations 20/min
(2)	3/20	ST segment elevation in II, III, and aVF
(3)	3/20	aPTT at 6 hours >120 seconds
(4)	3/20	aPTT at 12 hours 65 seconds
(5)	3/21	Urine output OK
(6)	3/22	Pulmonary rales, S_3
(7)	3/23	BP increased, patient appears irritable, anxious, heart rate 120
(8)	3/24	Appears well, good color, no chest pain, shortness of breath

88. From the medication orders written for Ms. Cunningham, it appears that captopril was prescribed shortly after the acute period of the heart attack. Based on the patient's profile, what is the most logical reason for including captopril in this setting?

    I. Adjunctive therapy to prevent left ventricular dysfunction after acute myocardial infarction
    II. Additive therapy to help bring the patient's blood pressure down
    III. Treatment of suspected renal dysfunction

    A. I only
    B. III only
    C. I and II
    D. II and III
    E. I, II, and III

89. The usual adult maintenance dose for levothyroxine is:

    A. 25–50 μg
    B. 100–200 μg
    C. 200–300 μg
    D. 400–500 μg
    E. 120 μg

90. On 3/23, Ms. Cunningham appears irritable. On examination, her heart rate is found to be 120, she is sweating profusely, and she has developed a noticeable tremor. Which drugs would most likely be contributing to these symptoms?

    I. Levothyroxine
    II. Amiodarone
    III. Captopril

    A. I only
    B. III only
    C. I and II
    D. II and III
    E. I, II, and III

91. The half-life of amiodarone is:

    A. 1 hour
    B. 6 hours
    C. 24 hours
    D. 50 hours
    E. Up to 50 days

92. Propranolol is administered to patients with hyperthyroidism because it:

    I. Helps to reduce tachycardia, sweating, and tremor associated with hyperthyroidism
    II. Inhibits the peripheral conversion of thyroxine (T_4) to triiodothyronine (T_3)
    III. Suppresses the production of T_4

    A. I only
    B. III only
    C. I and II
    D. II and III
    E. I, II, and III

93. Which of the following choices best summarize(s) the use of t-PA in the regimen used in the acute management of Ms. Cunningham's myocardial infarction?

    I. t-PA is the least expensive medication given when compared with streptokinase in the acute management of myocardial infarction.
    II. "Front-loaded" or "accelerated" t-PA to expedite opening of occluded coronary arteries
    III. The "open artery hypothesis" has been proven correct, and the earlier an infarcted artery is reopened after occlusion, the lower the mortality rate after an acute coronary occlusion and the better the long-term patency of the artery.

    A. I only
    B. III only
    C. I and II
    D. II and III
    E. I, II, and III

94. Atenolol is prescribed for the acute management of Ms. Cunningham's myocardial infarction for which of the following reasons?

    I. It is used as an adjunctive treatment that prevents angina pectoris and potentially significant atrial tachyarrhythmias.
    II. Atenolol is used in this patient to decrease the patient's blood pressure.
    III. β-adrenergic blockers have been shown to be effective in post-myocardial infarction patients in the prevention of mortality due to sudden cardiac death.

    A. I only
    B. III only
    C. I and II
    D. II and III
    E. I, II, and III

95. From the allergy history presented on admission by Ms. Cunningham, it appears that she has had some problems in the past taking quinidine as an antiarrhythmic. Are there ways to prevent these reactions?

    I. No, there has yet to be documented any method to desensitize the patient so that quinidine can be administered at a later date or time.
    II. Yes, administer aluminum hydroxide gel to prevent the reactions.
    III. Yes, the signs and symptoms reported reflect cinchonism, which can be prevented by reducing the dose of quinidine administered.

    A. I only
    B. III only
    C. I and II
    D. II and III
    E. I, II, and III

Use the patient profile below to answer questions 96–108.

MEDICATION PROFILE—COMMUNITY

Patient Name: Jon Rones
Address: 11 Cherry Lane
Age: 61   Height: 5'10"
Sex: M   Race: White   Weight: 230 lb
Allergies: Sulfonamides, penicillin; both cause rash

DIAGNOSIS
Primary   (1)   Acute renal failure
               (2)   Hyperkalemia
Secondary   (1)   Hypertension
               (2)   Heart failure
               (3)   Sinus congestion

MEDICATION RECORD Prescription and OTC

	Date	℞ No	Physician	Drug and Strength	Quan	Sig	Refills
(1)	6/8	245320	Sadler	Hydrochlorothiazide 50 mg	30	i qd	6
(2)	6/8	245321	Sadler	Moexipril 7.5 mg	30	i qd	6
(3)	6/8	245322	Sadler	Slow-K 8 mEq	100	i tid	6
(4)	6/15	246100	Frisch	Sudafed	100	i q 6 h	12
(5)	6/15	246101	Frisch	Tenuate Dospan	30	1 qd	5
(6)	11/7	278900	Sadler	Isoptin SR 120 mg	60	i bid	0
(7)	11/7	278901	Sadler	Tenormin 50 mg	60	i bid	0
(8)	11/7	278902	Sadler	Isordil 40 mg	120	i qid	5
(9)	11/7	278903	Sadler	Lanoxin 0.25 mg	30	i qd	0
(10)	12/5	279100	Frisch	Tenuate Dospan	30	i qd	5
(11)	2/5	280001	Sadler	Capoten 25 mg	100	i tid	1
(12)	2/5	280002	Sadler	Aldactone 25 mg	100	i tid	1
(13)	3/15	290016	Sadler	Vasotec 5 mg	60	i bid	6
(14)	3/15	290017	Sadler	Lanoxin 0.125 mg	30	i qd	6

PHARMACIST NOTES and Other Patient Information

	Date	Comments
(1)	11/7	D/C HydroDIURIL 50 mg
(2)	11/7	D/C Moexipril 7.5 mg
(3)	11/7	D/C Slow-K 8 mEq
(4)	2/5	D/C Lanoxin 0.25 mg
(5)	2/5	D/C Isoptin SR 120 mg
(6)	2/5	D/C Tenormin 50 mg
(7)	3/5	D/C Capoten 25 mg
(8)	3/5	D/C Aldactone 25 mg
(9)	3/5	D/C Sudafed
(10)	3/5	D/C Tenuate Dospan

96. Based on the patient's medication profile, which condition(s) are potential underlying causes of the acute renal failure in Mr. Rones?

    I. Heart failure
    II. Hypertension
    III. Hyperkalemia

    A. I only
    B. III only
    C. I and II
    D. II and III
    E. I, II, and III

97. Based on Mr. Rones's allergies, which medication can he receive safely?

    A. Hydrochlorothiazide
    B. V-Cillin-K
    C. Bactrim
    D. Septra
    E. None of the above

98. Based on the patient information, which medication would warrant a call to the physician before the pharmacist dispensed it to Mr. Rones?

    I. Slow-K
    II. Sudafed
    III. Moexipril

    A. I only
    B. III only
    C. I and II
    D. II and III
    E. I, II, and III

99. According to the Joint National Committee-7 guidelines, which agents are suitable alternatives to a thiazide diuretic for the initial treatment of Stage I hypertension in this patient?

    I. Atenolol
    II. Ramipril
    III. Candesartan

    A. I only
    B. III only
    C. I and II
    D. II and III
    E. I, II, and III

100. All of the following measures can be used in the prevention and treatment of digoxin-induced toxicity EXCEPT:

    A. Maintaining normal concentrations of potassium in the serum
    B. Routinely monitoring renal function to determine digoxin elimination
    C. Administering Kayexalate solutions
    D. Administering lidocaine
    E. None of the above

101. Which of the following choices accurately describes the agent listed and the drug class that it belongs to?

    I. Felodipine—β-adrenergic receptor blocker; ramipril—angiotensin-converting enzyme (ACE) inhibitor; losartan—calcium channel blocker; propranolol—β-adrenergic receptor blocker
    II. felodipine—calcium channel blocker; losartan—angiotensin II receptor antagonist; ramipril—ACE inhibitor; enalapril—ACE inhibitor
    III. atenolol—β-adrenergic receptor blocker; carvedilol—β-adrenergic receptor blocker; isradipine—calcium channel blocker; enalapril—ACE inhibitor

    A. I only
    B. III only
    C. I and II
    D. II and III
    E. I, II, and III

102. Which of the following would not be considered appropriate treatment for this patient's hyperkalemia?

    A. Dialysis
    B. Calcium chloride or calcium gluconate
    C. Regular insulin with dextrose
    D. Sodium polystyrene sulfonate
    E. Spironolactone

103. When dispensing the prescription for Isoptin and Tenormin, the pharmacist should advise Mr. Rones to:

    I. Check his heart rate regularly for brady-cardia.

    II. Report swelling, shortness of breath, and fatigue.

    III. Report orthopnea, dyspnea on exertion, and paroxysmal nocturnal dyspnea.

    A. I only
    B. III only
    C. I and II
    D. II and III
    E. I, II, and III

104. Which reference text could a pharmacist use to determine the indications and dosage for a relatively newly released medication for the treatment of hypertension?

    A. *Merck Index*
    B. American Hospital Formulary Service (AHFS)
    C. *Trissel's*
    D. *Hansten's*
    E. *Physicians' Desk Reference (PDR)*

105. The use of Lanoxin 0.125 mg for Mr. Rones centers around its ability to:

    A. Decrease the chronotropic actions of the heart, thereby reducing blood pressure
    B. Increase the chronotropic actions of the heart, thereby reducing blood pressure
    C. Increase renal blood flow, thereby improving urinary output
    D. Increase the inotropic actions of the heart, thereby increasing cardiac output
    E. Decrease the inotropic actions of the heart, thereby decreasing cardiac output

106. Digoxin has an elimination half-life of 36 hours and 4.5 days in patients who have normal renal function and in those who are anephric, respectively. If no loading doses were used in Mr. Rones and he is anephric, the time to reach steady-state serum digoxin concentrations would be approximately:

    A. 2–3 days
    B. 3–5 days
    C. 6–8 days
    D. 10–15 days
    E. 15–20 days

107. Which medication can be substituted for Inderal in a hypertensive patient who also suffers from bronchospastic lung disease and noncompliance?

    A. Inderal LA
    B. Blocadren
    C. Brevibloc
    D. Corgard
    E. Sectral

108. Which statements about the treatment of heart failure in Mr. Rones is/are correct?

    I. Isordil is probably being used as a preload reducing agent.

    II. Dopamine would be an appropriate alternative to Lanoxin in this patient.

    III. Dobutrex would be an appropriate alternative to Lanoxin in this patient.

    A. I only
    B. III only
    C. I and II
    D. II and III
    E. I, II, and III

End of this patient profile; continue with the examination

---

109. A patient has just returned from England, where she received a drug to treat her asthma. She asks for the United States equivalent for this drug. What is the best resource for identifying this drug?

    A. *Facts and Comparisons*
    B. *Martindale's Extra Pharmacopoeia*
    C. *Identidex*
    D. *Physicians' Desk Reference (PDR)*
    E. *Drug Information 1990*

110. Peritoneal dialysis is useful in removing drugs from an intoxicated person if the drug:

    A. is polar
    B. is lipid-soluble
    C. is highly bound to plasma proteins
    D. is nonpolar
    E. has a large apparent volume of distribution

111. Which of the following groups of herbal medicines are considered unsafe by the FDA due to their ability to cause damage to various organ systems?

    I. Tonka bean, heliotrope, and periwinkle, causing hepatotoxicity
    II. Mistletoe, spindle tree, and wahoo, causing seizures
    III. Jimson weed and sweet flag, causing hallucinations

    A. I only
    B. III only
    C. I and II
    D. II and III
    E. I, II, and III

112. The percentage of elemental iron in ferrous gluconate is:

    A. 10%
    B. 12%
    C. 20%
    D. 30%
    E. 33%

113. In the extemporaneous compounding of an ointment, the process of using a suitable nonsolvent to reduce the particle size of a drug before its incorporation into the ointment is known as:

    A. Geometric dilution
    B. Levigation
    C. Pulverization by intervention
    D. Spatulation
    E. Trituration

114. An antibiotic for IV infusion is supplied in 50-ml vials at a concentration of 5 mg/ml. How many vials are required for a 80-kg patient who needs an adult dose at a suggested infusion rate of 2.5 mg/kg/hr for 6 hours?

    A. 1
    B. 2
    C. 3
    D. 4
    E. 5

115. The bioavailability of a drug from an immediate-release tablet dosage form is most often related to the:

    A. Disintegration of the tablet
    B. Dissolution of the drug
    C. Elimination half-life of the drug
    D. Plasma protein binding of the drug
    E. Size of the tablet

116. Which of the following represents a list of protease inhibitors used in the treatment of human immunodeficiency virus (HIV)?

    I. Amprenavir, indinavir, and nelfinavir
    II. Zalcitabine, stavudine, lamivudine
    III. Delavirdine, efavirenz, nevirapine

    A. I only
    B. III only
    C. I and II
    D. II and III
    E. I, II, and III

117. The rate of dissolution of a weak acid drug may be increased by:

    I. Increasing the pH of the medium
    II. Increasing the particle size of the solid drug
    III. Increasing the viscosity of the medium

    A. I only
    B. III only
    C. I and II
    D. II and III
    E. I, II, and III

PATIENT RECORD—INSTITUTION/NURSING HOME

Patient Name: Bernard Hayley
Address: 2983 North Circle Dr
Age: 29   Height: 5'11"
Sex: M   Race: White   Weight: 200 lb
Allergies: Reaction to contrast media; hives

DIAGNOSIS
Primary   (1)   Bipolar affective disorder
               (2)
Secondary   (1)   Prehypertension (according to JNC-7)
               (2)   History of epilepsy

LAB/DIAGNOSTIC TESTS

	Date	Test		Date	Test
(1)	8/10	Lithium 0.9 mEq/L			
(2)	8/10	WBC 14,000 cells/mm³			

MEDICATION ORDERS Including Parenteral Solutions

	Date	Comments	Route	Sig
(1)	8/10	Lithium carbonate (Lithobid) 300 mg	po	i q 12 h
(2)	8/10	Tegretol 200 mg	po	i tid
(3)	8/10	Hydrochlorothiazide (HCTZ) 25 mg	po	i q AM
(4)	8/10	Ambien 10 mg	po	1 q hs prn
(5)	8/10	Acetaminophen 650 mg	po	i–ii q 4 h prn
(6)	8/10	May salt food as liberally as desired		

ADDITIONAL ORDERS

	Date	Comments
(1)		
(2)		

DIETARY CONSIDERATIONS Enteral and Parentral

	Date	Comments
(1)		
(2)		

PHARMACIST NOTES and Other Patient Information

	Date	Comments
(1)		
(2)		

118. Which statement concerning lithium is true?

   A. It is the drug of choice in the treatment and prophylaxis of manic episodes.
   B. It is classified as an anxiolytic.
   C. It is a serum electrolyte similar to sodium and is relatively free of serious adverse effects and drug interactions.
   D. It is commonly used as an antidepressant.
   E. It is similar to haloperidol in neuroleptic activity.

119. The molecular weight of lithium carbonate, Li_2CO_3, is 73.89. How many mEq of lithium are there in a 300-mg tablet of lithium carbonate?

   A. 1.24
   B. 2.46
   C. 4.06
   D. 8.12
   E. 12.18

120. The admitting physician had suspected that the patient was noncompliant with lithium therapy before admission. When interpreting the admission lithium level, the physician should consider:

    I. The sample "draw time" with respect to the time of the last scheduled lithium dose
    II. Concomitant drug therapy
    III. The acute manic condition of the patient

    A. I only
    B. III only
    C. I and II
    D. II and III
    E. I, II, and III

121. For monitoring this patient's serum lithium concentrations, the most consistent serum drug concentration that can be conveniently sampled is the:

    I. Minimum (trough) plasma drug concentration
    II. Average plasma drug concentration
    III. Peak plasma drug concentration

    A. I only
    B. III only
    C. I and II
    D. II and III
    E. I, II, and III

122. During the first 3 days of hospitalization, the patient has begun to exhibit a fine hand tremor and the symptoms of polyuria and polydipsia. Which statement would represent the most rational first step in management?

    A. The carbamazepine dose should be adjusted upward to control the hand tremor.
    B. A repeat lithium level should be obtained to assess therapy.
    C. The patient should be placed on an American Diabetes Association diet because he may be exhibiting signs and symptoms of diabetes mellitus.
    D. The effects are temporary and a saliva substitute may be needed.
    E. The patient's lithium therapy should be immediately decreased by one half because he is exhibiting a toxic reaction.

123. The hydrochlorothiazide order for Mr. Hayley might affect his serum lithium concentration by:

    A. Altering the glomerular filtration of lithium
    B. Increasing the absorption of lithium in the loop of Henle
    C. Increasing the absorption of lithium and sodium in the gastrointestinal tract
    D. Interfering with sodium reabsorption in the kidney
    E. Decreasing lithium reabsorption in the distal tubule

124. The physician has decided to add a selective serotonin reuptake inhibitor (SSRI) to the patient's treatment regimen. Which of the following choices best represents examples of these types of agents?

    I. Amitriptyline, doxepin, protriptyline
    II. Amoxapine, trazodone, bupropion
    III. Paroxetine, sertraline, fluoxetine

    A. I only
    B. III only
    C. I and II
    D. II and III
    E. I, II, and III

125. Based on Mr. Hayley's patient profile, if the physician were to initiate therapy with a tricyclic antidepressant, caution should be exercised with this patient because of which potentially life-threatening adverse effect?

    A. Mydriasis
    B. Tachycardia
    C. Dry mouth
    D. Lowered seizure threshold
    E. Systemic lupus erythematosus

126. If Mr. Hayley were started on an SSRI, what would be an "ideal" initial dose?

    A. Fluoxetine 10 mg q am
    B. Paroxetine 40 mg q pm
    C. Fluvoxamine 50 mg q am
    D. Sertraline 50 mg q pm

127. Which SSRI would have the greatest negative sexual side effects?

    A. Sertraline
    B. Fluvoxamine
    C. Fluoxetine
    D. Paroxetine

End of this patient profile; continue with the examination

---

128. Methotrexate is used alone or in combination for the treatment of various neoplastic diseases. A recommended IV loading dose of methotrexate for the treatment of acute lymphoblastic leukemia is 200 mg/m^2 (for the pediatric patient). What would be the loading dose for an 8-year-old patient whose body surface area is 0.89 m^2?

    A. 224 mg
    B. 150 mg
    C. 178 mg
    D. 200 mg
    E. 295 mg

129. The diuretic action of furosemide is due to:

    A. Osmotic activity within the renal tubules
    B. Inhibition of sodium and chloride reabsorption at the distal segment of the nephron
    C. Inhibition of carbonic anhydrase at the nephron
    D. Inhibition of sodium reabsorption at the ascending limb of the loop of Henle
    E. Inhibition of aldosterone at the distal segment of the nephron

130. Nonprescription decongestants used for topical application to the nasal passages include:

    I. Phenylephrine
    II. Xylometazoline
    III. Pseudoephedrine

    A. I only
    B. III only
    C. I and II
    D. II and III
    E. I, II, and III

131. According to the Joint National Committee-7, first-line drugs in the treatment of Stage 1 hypertension, in the absence of other disease states, include:

    I. Diuril
    II. Tenormin
    III. Catapres

    A. I only
    B. III only
    C. I and II
    D. II and III
    E. I, II, and III

132. To minimize the risk of tardive dyskinesia in a patient receiving antipsychotic drug therapy, the patient should be:

    I. Given the lowest possible doses of antipsychotic agents
    II. Monitored closely for symptoms of tardive dyskinesia
    III. Given a holiday from antipsychotic agents for a short period of time

    A. I only
    B. III only
    C. I and II
    D. II and III
    E. I, II, and III

133. Which of these agents would produce a significant drug–drug interaction in a patient who is taking Parnate?

    I. Demerol
    II. Morphine
    III. Ketorolac

    A. I only
    B. III only
    C. I and II
    D. II and III
    E. I, II, and III

134. Which agent is a selective antagonist of serotonin and has been shown to prevent the nausea and vomiting caused by highly emetogenic cancer chemotherapy?

    A. Zyban
    B. Zoloft
    C. Zyvox
    D. Zofran
    E. Zocor

135. Which of the following drugs is an antipsychotic agent?

    A. Aripiprazole
    B. Rabeprazole
    C. Butoconazole
    D. Clotrimazole

136. Which vitamin or other agent is often given along with a calcium supplement to aid in its absorption?

    A. Citracal
    B. Vitamin D
    C. Ascorbic acid
    D. Vitamin E
    E. Pantothenic Acid

137. All of the following would be good recommendations to prevent poison ivy contact dermatitis EXCEPT:

    A. Wash hands with soap and water within 10 minutes of exposure to poison ivy.
    B. Apply bentoquatam 5% solution at least 15 minutes before possible plant contact.
    C. Apply bentoquatam 5% solution immediately after contact with the poison ivy plant to exposed area of skin.
    D. Avoid the poison ivy plant.
    E. Identify the poison ivy plant in books, on TV, etc. so the patient will know what it looks like and how to avoid it.

Use the patient profile below to answer questions 138–148.

MEDICATION PROFILE—COMMUNITY

Patient Name: Barbara Szymuniak
Address: 200 Hawkins Dr
Age: 46
Sex: F
Race: White
Height: 5'10"
Weight: 150 lb
Allergies: Penicillin, codeine

DIAGNOSIS

Primary	(1)	Community-acquired pneumonia
	(2)	Rheumatoid arthritis
Secondary	(1)	Peptic ulcer disease
	(2)	Drug-induced duodenal ulcer
	(3)	

MEDICATION RECORD Prescription and OTC

	Date	℞ No	Physician	Drug and Strength	Quan	Sig	Refills
(1)	1/5	209356	Cook	Aspirin 325 mg	120	iii qid	0
(2)	1/5	209357	Cook	Cefaclor 250 mg	20	i PO bid	0
(3)	1/5	209360	Cook	Clarithromycin 500 mg	20	i PO bid	0
(4)	1/15	210200	Cook	Aspirin 325 mg	30	iv qid	0
(5)	1/21	210855	Smithson	Vitamin B_{12} 50 mg	30	i q AM	3
(6)	1/21	210856	Smithson	Folic acid 1 mg	30	i q AM	3
(7)	1/21	210857	Smithson	Ferrous sulfate 325 mg	30	i q tid	3
(8)	1/25	211324	Cook	Tagamet 300 mg	120	i tid	2
(9)	1/25	211325	Cook	Ecotrin 325 mg	120	iv qid	1
(10)	2/4	212003	Smithson	Cytotec 100 mg	120	i qid	6
(11)	2/4	212004	Smithson	Maalox Suspension	360	1 tsp qid	6
(12)	2/8	213344	Cook	Motrin 800 mg	90	i tid	3
(13)	3/1	215092	Cook	Cytotec 200 mg	120	i qid	3
(14)	4/1	216094	Cook	Celebrex 100 mg	60	i bid	
(15)	4/1	216095	Cook	Prevacid 15 mg	30	i PO q AM	3
(16)	5/1	220346	Cook	Enbrel 25 mg SQ	60	Twice weekly	3

PHARMACIST NOTES and Other Patient Information

	Date	Comments
(1)	1/25	D/C Aspirin; no benefit, GI intolerance
(2)	2/8	D/C Ecotrin; GI bleeding, anemia
(3)	3/1	D/C Tagamet
(4)	4/1	D/C Motrin; treat duodenal ulcer, drug-induced
(5)	5/1	D/C Prevacid; effective treatment of peptic ulcer disease
(6)	5/1	D/C Maalox Suspension

138. Which of the agents listed in the patient profile is a macrolide antibiotic?

    I. Cefaclor
    II. Celebrex
    III. Clarithromycin

    A. I only
    B. III only
    C. I and II
    D. II and III
    E. I, II, and III

139. All of the following medications can be crushed before swallowing EXCEPT:

    A. Aspirin
    B. Prilosec
    C. Plaquenil
    D. Motrin
    E. Tagamet

140. Which of the following choices best describes the action of Enbrel, which is currently being used in Ms. Szymuniak?

    I. It is a biological response modifier for slowing the progression of rheumatoid arthritis.
    II. It is an agent that inhibits only the cyclooxygenase-2 receptor and is effective in the treatment of rheumatoid arthritis.
    III. It is an inhibitor of both cyclooxygenase-2 and -1 receptors and is indicated in the treatment of symptoms associated with rheumatoid arthritis.

    A. I only
    B. III only
    C. I and II
    D. II and III
    E. I, II, and III

141. Which medication below, which may be used in the treatment of rheumatoid arthritis, requires close monitoring by an ophthalmologist to prevent adverse effects on the eyes?

    I. Motrin
    II. Celebrex
    III. Plaquenil

    A. I only
    B. III only
    C. II and III
    D. I, II, and III

142. All of the following agents could be used to replace Plaquenil EXCEPT:

    A. Plavix
    B. Ridaura
    C. Rheumatrex
    D. Depen
    E. Myochrysine

143. Which agents would be appropriate alternatives to the use of Motrin for Ms. Szymuniak?

    I. Celebrex
    II. Naprosyn
    III. Nabumetone

    A. III only
    B. I and II
    C. I only
    D. II and III
    E. I, II, and III

144. Which adverse drug reactions should be monitored in a patient receiving hydroxychloroquine?

    I. Visual changes
    II. Agranulocytosis
    III. Hemolytic anemia

    A. I only
    B. III only
    C. I and II
    D. II and III
    E. I, II, and II

145. Which of the following brand name/generic name NSAID listings match?

    I. Lodine/sulindac
    II. Vioxx/celecoxib
    III. Naprosyn/naproxen

    A. I only
    B. III only
    C. I and II
    D. II and III
    E. I, II, and III

146. Aspirin in high doses follows Michaelis-Menton kinetics, which describes:

    I. First-order elimination pharmacokinetics
    II. Nonlinear pharmacokinetics
    III. Maximum velocity (V_{max}) and Km of enzyme kinetics

    A. I only
    B. III only
    C. I and II
    D. II and III
    E. I, II, and III

147. The prescriptions that Dr. Smithson wrote for Ms. Szymuniak on 1/21 were most likely given for:

    I. Tinnitus caused by high-dose aspirin therapy
    II. Renal parenchymal damage from long-term, high-dose aspirin therapy
    III. Gastrointestinal damage caused by long-term, high-dose aspirin therapy

    A. I only
    B. III only
    C. I and II
    D. II and III
    E. I, II, and III

148. Which presenting complaints associated with rheumatoid arthritis are correct?

    I. Morning stiffness in and around the joint lasting at least 1 hour before improvement
    II. Presentation of subcutaneous nodules over bony prominences or extensor surfaces
    III. Asymmetric involvement of the body joints

    A. I only
    B. III only
    C. I and II
    D. II and III
    E. I, II, and III

End of this patient profile; continue with the examination

---

149. Unfractionated heparin (UFH) blocks coagulation by inactivating which of the following clotting factors?

    I. Factor IIa
    II. Factor Xa
    III. Factor IXa

    A. I only
    B. III only
    C. I and II
    D. II and III
    E. I, II and III

150. Sally, a regular customer in your pharmacy, wants some advice on an OTC treatment for itchy, odorous feet. Upon questioning, you discover that in between her toes, the skin is whiter than usual, thick, and scaly. She tells you that she swims competitively and often uses public showers at the pool. What condition is Sally most likely suffering from?

    A. Tinea cruris
    B. Tinea capitis
    C. Tinea pedis
    D. Tinea corporis
    E. Tinea unguium

151. All of the following OTC agents below are considered safe and effective for treating Sally's condition (question #150) EXCEPT:

    A. Terbinafine
    B. Clotrimazole
    C. Tolnaftate
    D. Hexylresorcinol
    E. Miconazole

152. What are the two OTC antihistamines approved by the FDA for insomnia?

    A. Diphenhydramine and doxylamine
    B. Chlorpheniramine and loratadine
    C. Doxylamine and brompheniramine
    D. Thonzylamine and pheniramine
    E. Dexbrompheniramine and chlorpheniramine

153. Mr. Conway, a 45-year-old man who drives cross-country for a trucking company, complains of a runny nose, sneezing, and watery eyes that typically occur about this time of year. He knows it is allergies but cannot remember what medication he took for his allergies last year. Which of the following would be the best initial OTC recommendation for Mr. Conway to take for this condition this year?

    A. Pseudoephedrine 30 mg BID
    B. Loratadine 10 mg QD
    C. Diphenhydramine 25 mg q6h
    D. No OTC recommendation; refer the patient to a physician for an Rx for a nonsedating antihistamine

154. On a slow Sunday afternoon, you spot a young woman in the analgesic aisle and ask if there's anything you can help her find. She blushes a bit and blurts, "I just started my period and I think I'm going to die if I don't take something pretty quick here!" You hide your surprise (after all, this is a 12-year-old daughter of one of your friends at church) and offer to help. Which of the following medications is NOT an option for this patient?

    A. Ketoprofen
    B. Acetaminophen
    C. Ibuprofen
    D. Naproxen
    E. Aspirin

155. Your pharmacy student pulls you aside and asks, "I'm trying to counsel Mrs. Pound on the nonprescription medication treatment options to take care of her daughter's head lice." Which of the following products could be recommended?

    I. A synergized pyrethrins product
    II. A product containing permethrin
    III. A product containing lindane

    A. I only
    B. III only
    C. I and II
    D. II and III
    E. I, II, and III

156. There are a large number of insulin products. Novolin 70/30 is composed of which of the following?

    A. 70% Regular insulin, 30% NPH insulin
    B. 70% Humalog insulin, 30% NPH insulin
    C. 70% NPH insulin, 30% Regular insulin
    D. 70% NPH insulin, 30% Humalog insulin

Use the patient profile below to answer questions 157–168.

MEDICATION PROFILE—COMMUNITY

Patient Name: _Fanny Urmeister_
Address: _24555 Colonial Estates_
Age: _79_   Height: _5'2"_
Sex: _F_   Race: _Black_   Weight: _178 lb_
Allergies: _Aspirin_

DIAGNOSIS
Primary   (1)   Arrhythmias
               (2)
Secondary   (1)   Status post NSTEMI
               (2)   Smoking
               (3)   Obesity

MEDICATION RECORD Prescription and OTC

	Date	℞ No	Physician	Drug and Strength	Quan	Sig	Refills
(1)	10/5	111345	Lamb	Tambocor 50 mg	60	i bid	6
(2)	10/5	111346	Lamb	Docusate 100 mg	60	ii hs	6
(3)	10/5	111347	Lamb	Ecotrin 325 mg	30	i q AM	6
(4)	10/5	111348	Lamb	Coumadin 2.5 mg	30	i q AM	6
(5)	10/5	111349	Troys	Nicoderm Patches	1	ut dict	0
(6)	10/26	111941	Troys	Procan SR 500 mg	60	i qid	6
(7)	10/26	111942	Lamb	Isordil 20 mg	120	i q 6 h	3
(8)	11/2	112300	Cold	Isuprel Inhalation	1	ut dict	4
(9)	11/2	112301	Cold	Dimetane 4 mg	30	i q 8 h	0
(10)	11/5	112589	Lamb	Quinidex 300 mg	60	i q 8 h	6
(11)	11/5	112590	Lamb	Robitussin-DM	120	i tsp q 4 h	0
(12)	11/5	112591	Lamb	Imodium 2 mg	30	ut dict	0

PHARMACIST NOTES and Other Patient Information

	Date	Comments
(1)	10/26	D/C Tambocor
(2)	11/5	D/C Procan SR
(3)	11/5	D/C Imodium

157. Based on Ms. Urmeister's allergies, which medications may be filled by the pharmacist?

    I. Tambocor

    II. Coumadin

    III. Ecotrin

    A. I only

    B. III only

    C. I and II

    D. II and III

    E. I, II, and III

158. Which medications best represent class I antiarrhythmics?

    I. Quinidine, procainamide, and disopyramide

    II. Lidocaine, tocainide, and mexiletine

    III. Flecainide, propafenone, and moricizine

    A. I only

    B. III only

    C. I and II

    D. II and III

    E. I, II, and III

159. What are the advantages of Procan SR tablets over Pronestyl capsules?

    I. Procan SR tablets provide more procainamide per dose.
    II. Procan SR tablets are taken less frequently.
    III. After Procan SR treatment, the plasma procainamide hydrochloride levels have smaller fluctuations between peak and trough levels.

    A. I only
    B. III only
    C. I and II
    D. II and III
    E. I, II, and III

160. Which medications would be appropriate for Ms. Urmeister during the first several hours after her myocardial infarction?

    I. Reteplase
    II. Metoprolol
    III. Heparin

    A. I only
    B. III only
    C. I and II
    D. II and III
    E. I, II, and III

161. Which treatments for Ms. Urmeister are likely to include Isordil?

    I. Treatment of heart failure after a myocardial infarction
    II. Treatment of the increased oxygen demand causing angina pectoris
    III. Acute treatment of hypertension

    A. I only
    B. III only
    C. I and II
    D. II and III
    E. I, II, and III

162. Which choices may result in increased oxygen demand by the myocardium and, therefore, may cause a problem in Ms. Urmeister?

    I. Isoproterenol
    II. Smoking
    III. Acebutolol

    A. I only
    B. III only
    C. I and II
    D. II and III
    E. I, II, and III

163. The physician would like the pharmacist to dispense a generic drug product that is bioequivalent to Quinidex. This generic drug product should have:

    I. The same drug bioavailability
    II. An equal or better rate and extent of systemic drug absorption
    III. An equal or better C_{max}, area under the curve (AUC), and T_{max}

    A. I only
    B. III only
    C. I and II
    D. II and III
    E. I, II, and III

164. Which agent would be a suitable first-line oral drug to use in this patient, who needs maintenance therapy for ventricular tachycardia?

    A. Tambocor
    B. Enkaid
    C. Lidocaine
    D. Tikosyn
    E. Mexitil

165. Which agents that Ms. Urmeister has received are most likely to be responsible for her use of Imodium on 11/5?

    I. Tambocor
    II. Procan SR
    III. Quinidex

    A. I only
    B. III only
    C. I and II
    D. II and III
    E. I, II, and III

166. Which agent is effective in reducing pain, anxiety, and cardiac workload in the myocardial infarction patient?

    A. Aspirin
    B. Morphine
    C. Furosemide
    D. Digoxin
    E. Lidocaine

167. Which agents are effective in preventing sudden death in post-myocardial infarction patients?

    I. Procan SR
    II. Blocadren
    III. Tenormin

    A. I only
    B. III only
    C. I and II
    D. II and III
    E. I, II, and III

168. All of the following generic/brand-name combinations are correct EXCEPT:

    A. Quinidine sulfate (Quinidex)
    B. Warfarin (Coumadin)
    C. Nitroglycerin patches (Nicoderm Patches)
    D. Disopyramide (Norpace)
    E. Diltiazem (Cardizem)

169. A 30-year-old male comes into your pharmacy complaining of difficulty falling asleep at night. He hands you a list of all the drugs he is currently taking. Which one of these medications is the most likely culprit responsible for this sleep problem?

    A. Metamucil
    B. Sudafed
    C. Flonase
    D. Benadryl
    E. Aspirin

170. Which of the following conditions can be treated with nonprescription products?

    A. Water-clogged ears
    B. Otitis media
    C. Swimmer's Ear
    D. Impacted cerumen
    E. Both A & D

171. Which of the following topical nasal decongestant agents has a 12-hour duration of action and, therefore, is administered twice daily for adult patients?

    A. oxymetazoline
    B. naphazoline
    C. phenylephrine
    D. ephedrine
    E. propylhexedrine

172. Jim, a technician working in your pharmacy, asks you to recommend a sunscreen for him to take to the beach for spring break. He has fair skin and states that he usually burns after only 10 minutes in the sun. If you recommend an SPF of 15 and you assume Jim applies this product correctly, how many minutes will Jim be protected?

    A. 30 minutes
    B. 2 hours 30 minutes
    C. 6 hours
    D. 45 minutes
    E. 1 hour and 30 minutes

173. A 21-year-old male walks up to you at the counter with a bottle of 5% minoxidil in hand. He proceeds to ask you about how to effectively apply this product. All of the following are appropriate points to cover in counseling this patient EXCEPT:

     A. Double the dose if you miss an application.
     B. Apply or spray about 1 ml of the product onto the affected area of the scalp twice daily.
     C. This strength is only indicated for men, not women.
     D. This product must be used continuously to maintain any hair regrowth.
     E. Allow 4 hours for the drug to penetrate the scalp before showering or going swimming.

174. Which of the following nonprescription ingredients/combination of ingredients does NOT have proven safety/efficacy for the treatment of acne?

     A. Benzoyl peroxide
     B. Sulfur
     C. Triclosan
     D. Salicylic acid
     E. Sulfur and resorcinol

175. A teenage girl and her mother are at your counseling window in the pharmacy. The mother explains that her daughter has had acne for a few months now and has used a couple of OTC agents (benzoyl peroxide cream and face wash), and asks you to recommend a product to help treat the acne. You examine the girl's face and count over a dozen papules and pustules along with some mild scarring. She says she has a few more on her trunk.

     What would you recommend for this patient?

     A. Oxy Balance Deep Action Night Formula® (benzoyl peroxide 2.5%) each evening
     B. Clearasil Clearstick Maximum Strength® (salicylic acid 2%) each morning
     C. Wash face at least 4–5 times daily with SAStid Soap® (precipitated sulfur 10%)
     D. No further OTC product recommendations at this time; advise mother to take daughter to a physician or dermatologist
     E. Wash face no more than twice daily with a product such as Oxy 10 Balance Maximum Medicated Face Wash® (benzoyl peroxide 10%)

176. Which one of the following BEST describes the mechanism of action of benzoyl peroxide for acne?

     A. Porolytic—allows the pores to "open up"
     B. Keratolytic only
     C. Antibacterial only
     D. Releases oxygen to destroy the anaerobic *P. acnes;* and peeling outer layer of skin
     E. Dries out lesions by decreasing sebum production by sebaceous glands

177. Rhinitis Medicamentosa is an adverse effect associated with overuse of which agents?

    A. Oral decongestants
    B. Antihistamines
    C. Topical decongestants
    D. Expectorants
    E. Cough suppressants

178. The pharmacist should advise a patient not to crush Tenuate Dospan because crushing this tablet:

    I. Destroys the active drug in this dosage form
    II. Allows immediate absorption of the active drug
    III. Destroys the integrity of the delivery system

    A. I only
    B. III only
    C. I and II
    D. II and III
    E. I, II, and III

179. A first-order reaction is characterized by:

    I. $\frac{da}{dt} = -k$
    II. $A = A_0e^{-kt}$
    III. $t_{1/2} = \frac{0.693}{k}$

    A. I only
    B. III only
    C. I and II
    D. II and III
    E. I, II, and III

180. Flumist is approved for use in:

    I. Children ages 6 months–<5 years
    II. Children ages 5–17
    III. Adults ages 18–49

    A. I only
    B. III only
    C. I and II
    D. II and III
    E. I, II, and III

181. Calcium is available for oral administration in all of the following salt forms EXCEPT:

    A. Chloride
    B. Lactate
    C. Gluconate
    D. Phosphate
    E. Carbonate

182. All of the following are side effects of prednisone EXCEPT:

    A. Osteonecrosis
    B. Hyperglycemia
    C. Leukopenia
    D. Fluid retention
    E. Cataracts

183. Which of the following is NOT a protease inhibitor for treatment of HIV infection?

    A. Saquinavir
    B. Ritonavir
    C. Cidofovir
    D. Indinavir
    E. Crixivan

184. Pyrogen testing of parenteral solutions is a quality control procedure used to check that:

    I. The product does not contain fever-producing substances.
    II. The product is sterile.
    III. The product does not contain particulate matter.

    A. I only
    B. III only
    C. I and II
    D. II and III
    E. I, II, and III

185. Common laboratory tests to assess kidney disease include:

    I. Blood urea nitrogen (BUN) and serum creatinine
    II. Lactic dehydrogenase (LDG), aspartate aminotransferase (AST, formerly SGOT), and alanine aminotransferase (ALT, formerly SGPT)
    III. Red blood count (RBC) and white blood count (WBC)

    A. I only
    B. III only
    C. I and II
    D. II and III
    E. I, II, and III

186. Treatment of chemotherapy-induced nausea and vomiting includes all of the following drugs EXCEPT:

    A. Zofran
    B. Reglan
    C. Inapsine
    D. Tagamet
    E. Marinol

187. Laboratory findings in acute renal failure include all of the following conditions EXCEPT:

    A. Hypophosphatemia
    B. Hyperuricemia
    C. Hyperkalemia
    D. Metabolic acidosis
    E. Hypocalcemia

188. Which trace element, if deficient, is responsible for cretinism in children?

    A. Zinc
    B. Copper
    C. Chromium
    D. Selenium
    E. Iodine

189. All of the following are true of omalizumab EXCEPT:

    A. It is an immunoglobulin (Ig) monoclonal antibody that blocks the IgE receptor and thereby decreases allergic reactions.
    B. It is administered orally bid.
    C. It is approved for adults and adolescents with steroid-resistant asthma.
    D. It requires refrigeration during storage.
    E. Benefits may take several weeks to be noticeable.

End of this patient profile; End of Exam 1

TEST I ANSWERS AND EXPLANATIONS

1. The answer is E (I, II, and III).
The two potential problems included (1) the drug interaction between niacin and atorvastatin and (2) the use of aspirin in a patient with a history of an aspirin allergy. The combination of niacin and atorvastatin may increase the risk of myopathy and rhabdomyolysis (additive effects) and should be brought to the prescriber's attention. Aspirin is contraindicated in patients who are hypersensitive to it, as stated in Ms. Sprints' profile.

2. The answer is A.
Doxazosin in doses of 2 to 8 mg/day was one of the treatment arms in the recent Antihypertensive and Lipid-Lowering Treatment to Prevent Heart Attack Trial (ALLHAT), and the treatment was discontinued prematurely due to an apparent 25% increase in the incidence of combined cardiovascular disease outcomes compared to patients in the control group receiving the diuretic chlorthalidone. The added risks for heart failure, stroke, and coronary heart disease were the major outcomes affected in the doxazosin arm. The Heart Outcomes Prevention Evaluation (HOPE) project was one of the first clinical trials demonstrating the benefits of angiotensin-converting enzyme inhibitors (ramipril) in reducing cardiovascular death, myocardial infarction, and stroke in patients who were at high risk for or had vascular disease in the absence of heart failure. Ramipril, in doses of 10 mg per day, demonstrated substantial clinical benefits that could not be explained through its blood pressure-lowering effects alone.

3. The answer is E (I, II, and III).
The JNC-7 provided a table of "compelling" indications that suggested specific drug therapy in select patients rather the use of standard suggested guidelines. Included as compelling indications, and their respective therapy, are heart failure (diuretics, β-blockers, ACE inhibitors, angiotensin II receptor blockers [ARB], aldosterone antagonist), post-myocardial infarction (β-blockers, ACE inhibitors, aldosterone antagonist), high coronary disease risk (diuretics, β-blockers, ACE inhibitors, calcium channel blockers), diabetes (diuretics, β-blockers, ACE inhibitors, ARB, calcium channel blockers), chronic kidney disease (ACE inhibitors, ARB), and recurrent stroke prevention (diuretics, ACE inhibitors).

4. The answer is C (I and II).
β-adrenergic blockers such as atenolol are now indicated in patients post-MI, in whom they have been shown to significantly reduce sudden death and overall mortality. Additionally, they have been suggested by the JNC-7 guidelines as therapeutic options in hypertensive patients with the following "compelling" indications for their use instead of standard suggested therapy: congestive heart failure, post-MI, high-risk coronary disease patients, and diabetes. Ms. Sprints, as a post-MI patient with hypertension, would be a candidate for atenolol.

5. The answer is E (I, II, and III).
Thrombolytic agents (t-PA, r-PA, APSAC, SK, TNK) have been used in patients with STEMI who have had chest pain for less than 6 to 12 hours. Successful early reperfusion has been shown to reduce infarct size, improve ventricular function, and improve mortality. Benefits may be seen in patients using thrombolytic therapy as late as 12 hours after pain starts. The use of thrombolytics may restore blood flow in an occluded artery if administered within 12 hours of an acute MI, although less than 6 hours is optimal. The goal of treatment of STEMI patients is to initiate thrombolytic therapy within 30 to 60 minutes of arrival in an emergency room. Though which agent—t-PA, SK, APSAC, r-PA, and TNK—is best is still controversial, most studies have shown that each agent, when used early, can reopen (reperfuse) occluded coronary arteries and reduce mortality from STEMI. However, considerations such as ease of use, onset of action, incidence of bleed, and cost are important factors in determining which agent is used in a given hospital and patient.

6. The answer is C (I, II).
Clopidogrel is a thienopyridine derivative related to ticlopidine but possesses antithrombotic effects that are greater than those of ticlopidine. Clopidogrel is a therapeutic option in patients who cannot take aspirin due to contraindications. A dosage of 75 mg daily is recommended to prevent the development of acute coronary syndromes.

7. The answer is B.
Rabeprazole is a proton pump inhibitor (PPI), which among other indications (gastroesophageal reflux disease, erosive gastritis, hypersecretory conditions, and treatment of *Helicobacter pylori* infections) is also indicated for the treatment of duodenal ulcer. Rabeprazole is one of five currently available PPIs; the others are esomeprazole, lansoprazole, omeprazole, and pantoprazole. Current recommendations suggest a dosage of 20 mg by mouth daily for 4 weeks, which may be repeated for an additional 4 weeks if needed.

8. The answer is B (III only).
Sublingual nitroglycerin is indicated for the acute treatment of angina pectoris as well as for the pro-phylaxis of angina pectoris. The tablets are to be placed under the tongue, where they dissolve and demonstrate a quick onset of action of about 2 to 5 minutes. Sublingual nitroglycerin tablets are not to be swallowed or placed in easy-to-open plastic containers and should remain in the manufacturer's bottle to reduce loss of potency. Patients should also be warned that they may become light-headed or dizzy after taking a tablet and should either sit down or support themselves against a solid object to prevent falls. Patients should also be informed that nitroglycerin tablets can cause a headache and rou-tinely cause a slight burning sensation when placed under the tongue.

9. The answer is C.
JNC-7 guidelines include four blood pressure classes (normal, prehypertension, Stage I hypertension, and Stage II hypertension); the classes are based on patient blood pressure readings and are linked to current treatment recommendations. Normal (systolic <120 and diastolic <80 mm Hg) requires no treatment. Prehypertension (systolic 120 to 139 or diastolic of 80 to 89 mm Hg) again requires no an-tihypertensive treatment unless the patient has a compelling indication. In Stage I hypertension (systolic 140 to 159 or diastolic 90 to 99 mm Hg), thiazide-type diuretics are indicated for most patients, though patients with compelling indications would be candidates for other agents. In Stage II hypertension (sys-tolic ≥160 or diastolic ≥100 mm Hg), two-drug combinations are indicated for most patients (thiazide-type diuretic and ACE inhibitor, ARB, or β-blocker, or calcium channel blocker). Ms. Sprints currently is receiving a diuretic, a β-blocker, and an ACE inhibitor and is most likely considered to have Stage II hypertension.

10. The answer is E.
The patient profile states that the patient has an allergy to aspirin, which has resulted in an anaphylac-tic reaction. Consequently, all salicylates such as salsalate would be contraindicated. Additionally, all NSAIDs (ibuprofen-like as well as the newer COX-2 selective agents such as celecoxib, meloxicam, and rofecoxib) are contraindicated and should not be given to this patient.

11. The answer is E (I, II, and III).
Untreated hypertension has been shown to cause target organ damage to four major organ systems. Car-diac effects—left ventricular hypertrophy compensates for the increased cardiac workload, resulting in signs and symptoms of heart failure, and increased oxygen requirements of the enlarged heart may pro-duce angina pectoris. Hypertension can be caused by accelerated atherosclerosis. Atheromatous lesions in the coronary arteries lead to decreased blood flow, resulting in angina pectoris and myocardial in-farction and sudden death may ensue. Renal effects—decreased blood flow leads to an increase in renin-aldosterone secretion, which heightens the reabsorption of sodium and water and increases blood vol-ume. Accelerated atherosclerosis decreases the oxygen supply, leading to renal parenchymal damage, with decreased filtration capability, and azotemia. The atherosclerosis also decreases blood flow to the renal arterioles, leading to nephrosclerosis and, ultimately, renal failure (acute as well as chronic). Cere-bral effects—decreased blood flow, decreased oxygen supply, and weakened blood vessel walls lead to transient ischemic attacks, cerebral thromboses, and the development of aneurysms with hemorrhage. There are alterations in mobility, weakness and paralysis, and memory deficits. Retinal effects—decreased blood flow with retinal vascular sclerosis and increased arteriolar pressure with the appear-ance of exudates and hemorrhage result in visual defects (e.g., blurred vision, spots, blindness).

12. The answer is A.
In an otherwise healthy patient with Stage I hypertension, thiazide diuretics are considered the first-line treatment of choice for most patients. In patients who might have a compelling indication such as re-nal disease, stroke, high-risk cardiovascular disease, or diabetes mellitus, other agents have been rec-ommended. Amiloride is referred to as a potassium-sparing diuretic that inhibits distal convoluted

tubule aldosterone-induced sodium resorption and is not generally indicated over thiazide diuretics as first-line therapy. Chlorthalidone, chlorothiazide, indapamide, and methyclothiazide are all thiazide diuretics, and though they may have different pharmacokinetic profiles and different costs, they should all be considered first-line antihypertensives.

13. The answer is A (I).
IV infusion and a few controlled-release drug products provide zero-order drug absorption. The main advantage of zero-order absorption is to provide plasma drug concentrations that do not fluctuate widely between peak and trough levels. Plasma drug concentrations with wide fluctuations may rise above or below the therapeutic window for the drug.

14. The answer is A (I).
The mechanism of action of H_2-receptor antagonists is to decrease gastric acid secretion by inhibiting histamine at parietal receptor sites. Sucralfate, by contrast, forms a protective barrier against acid at the ulcer site. Anticholinergic agents act by decreasing gastrointestinal motility.

15. The answer is E (I, II, and III).
Insulin resistance is defined as the need for more than 200 U of insulin per day in the absence of ketoacidosis. Causes include obesity, infection, glucocorticoid therapy, and circulating IgG anti-insulin antibodies. Insulin resistance may resolve without treatment, by insulin switching, or with prednisone therapy.

16. The answer is C (I, II).
Lanolin (hydrous wool fat) has been used as an emulsion base where occlusive films can prevent water loss from the skin through evaporation.

17. The answer is D (II, III).
Kaopectate and Pepto-Bismol are considered effective in the treatment of diarrhea. Donnagel-PG is an opiate-containing antidiarrheal that exerts a direct musculotropic effect, which inhibits propulsive intestinal movements. Its value as an antidiarrheal is unproven. Both Kaopectate (attapulgite) and Pepto-Bismol (bismuth salts) are considered adsorbents, which are nonabsorbable inert powders that adsorb bacteria, toxins, and gases.

18. The answer is A (I).
Dopamine does not cross the blood–brain barrier, but its precursor levodopa does. Levodopa is metabolized centrally and peripherally to dopamine by dopa-decarboxylase. Carbidopa does not cross the blood–brain barrier and inhibits peripheral decarboxylation of levodopa. Therefore, more levodopa is available for transport to the brain, and the peripheral side effects are reduced. Sinemet combines the antiparkinsonian effects of levodopa with the dopamine metabolism-inhibiting effects of carbidopa.

19. The answer is C (I, II).
The only approved OTC stimulant is caffeine, which is available in NoDoz, Vivarin, and Dexitac. Dexatrim is an OTC appetite suppressant that contains phenylpropanolamine and is approved as a treatment for obesity.

20. The answer is A.
The action of salmeterol is that of a sympathomimetic agonist with high β_2 selectivity. The lung contains β_2 receptors, which are responsible for the relaxation of tracheal and bronchial muscles. In contrast, β_1 receptors are in the heart and are responsible for chronotropic (rate) and inotropic (contraction force) effects. Salmeterol gives the asthmatic patient maximal bronchodilation with minimal stimulation of cardiac receptors.

21. The answer is E (I, II, and III).
Varying age groups have common underlying causes for the development of heart failure. The patient in this case is 48 years of age, with a history of myocardial infarction as a possible etiology because it is a leading cause of heart failure in persons ages 40 to 50. Drugs such as corticosteroids also have been implicated as causative agents in the development of heart failure. In both of these cases, metabolic demands placed on the heart normally do not increase; however, the heart is still unable to meet

them (low output). Mr. Melvick has a secondary diagnosis of anemia (possibly caused by steroid use), which increases the metabolic demands placed on a heart that is already unable to meet such demands (high output).

22. The answer is B (III).

On receiving the prescription for enalapril (Vasotec) on 9/10, the pharmacist should have called the physician's office for assurance that the potassium supplement Slow-K was truly warranted in combination with the angiotensin-converting enzyme (ACE) inhibitor. ACE inhibitors may produce additive hyperkalemic effects when used with potassium supplements; therefore, use of this combination requires close monitoring of serum potassium to avoid toxicity. There is no real drug–drug interaction identified between the isosorbide dinitrate and hydralazine. The Veterans Administration study has shown that the combination of these two products had a positive effect on reducing mortality in patients not responsive to digoxin and diuretics.

23. The answer is D (II and III).

Carvedilol is a β-adrenergic receptor blocker that is indicated in the treatment of hypertension and heart failure. When used in the treatment of heart failure, as in Mr. Melvick, doses must be slowly titrated up to the maximal dosage every 2 weeks as tolerated. The pharmacist was able to identify that there were no prescriptions on file for Mr. Melvick for Coreg and there were no refills provided with the initial prescription of Coreg 3.125 mg. Cardiac patients receiving β-adrenergic receptor blockers should not have their β-blocker discontinued abruptly, as this may induce an acute coronary event due to the lack of β-blockade.

24. The answer is A.

A patient with left-sided heart failure would present with symptoms and signs of fluid backing up behind a failed left ventricle. Mr. Melvick would initially present with complaints involving the pulmonary system (e.g., rales, shortness of breath, paroxysmal nocturnal dyspnea). Peripheral signs and symptoms (e.g., jugular venous distention, hepatojugular reflux, pedal edema, abdominal distention, and hepatomegaly) are more the consequence of the backup of fluid behind the failing right ventricle, characteristically seen in right-sided heart failure. It is important to recognize that due to the closed system, which the circulatory system is, rarely do patients present with strictly left-sided signs or right-sided signs; rather, they present with a combination of signs and symptoms reflective of global circulatory problems.

25. The answer is C.

Altace or ramipril is an angiotensin-converting enzyme (ACE) inhibitor. Recent clinical guidelines recommend the use of ACE inhibitors in all patients with heart failure due to left ventricular systolic dysfunction unless they have a contraindication to their use or have demonstrated intolerance to their use. Currently, they are considered the first-line agents in the treatment of heart failure and have been shown to have a beneficial effect on cardiac remodeling. The Heart Outcomes Prevention Evaluation (HOPE) trial demonstrated that the ACE inhibitor ramipril (10 mg/day) reduced cardiovascular death, myocardial infarction, and stroke in patients older than 55 years of age who were at high risk for or had vascular disease in the absence of heart failure.

26. The answer is B.

Ferrous sulfate is available in the hydrous form as a 325-mg tablet. The preparation contains 20% elemental iron. Consequently, 325 mg given three times a day would equal $0.20 \times 3 \times 325$ mg, or 195 mg per day. Other available salts that contain varying degrees of elemental iron are ferrous gluconate, 12%; ferrous fumarate, 33%; and ferrous sulfate (desiccated), 30%.

27. The answer is C (I, II).

All diuretics are capable of reducing total body and sodium reabsorption through their diuretic effects on the kidney. These effects reduce venous return to the heart and decrease preload. Lasix (furosemide) has an additional benefit, in the acute situation, of causing a direct dilating effect on the lung, and it is a useful agent for the rapid reversal of pulmonary congestion. Current national guidelines recommend the use of a diuretic for patients with heart failure accompanied by fluid retention (edema), or those who have had fluid retention in the past with heart failure. Lasix has yet to show any significant effect on cytokines and their subsequent release.

28. The answer is C (I, II).
Enalapril (Vasotec), captopril (Capoten), lisinopril (Zestril and Prinivil), benazepril (Lotensin), fosinopril (Monopril), quinapril (Accupril), ramipril (Altace), moexipril (Univasc), and trandolapril (Mavik) are the angiotensin-converting enzyme (ACE) inhibitors currently on the market. The agents as a group have the same general pharmacologic effects by blocking the actions of the converting enzyme, which converts angiotensin I to angiotensin II (a potent vasoconstrictor, thereby reducing afterload, and stimulator of aldosterone release from the adrenal gland). Currently, ACE inhibitors are considered the first-line agents in the treatment of heart failure and have been shown to have a beneficial effect on cardiac remodeling.

29. The answer is D (II and III).
Digoxin molecules in tablet or capsule form have the same potency. The Lanoxicaps capsule is a liquid-filled capsule containing digoxin dissolved in a solvent composed of polyethylene glycol 400 USP, ethyl alcohol (8%), propylene glycol USP, and purified water. The systemic absorption of digoxin from the capsule is practically complete (F 90%–100%) and less variable than the systemic absorption of digoxin from the tablet (F 60%–80%). Digitalis, specifically digoxin, is now recommended in conjunction with diuretics, an ACE inhibitor, and a β-adrenergic blocker to improve the symptoms and clinical status of patients with heart failure due to left ventricular systolic dysfunction.

30. The answer is A.
Hydralazine (Apresoline) is an arteriolar dilator that has been used in hypertension. However, by decreasing peripheral vascular resistance, it also has been shown to reduce afterload in patients with heart failure. The Veterans Administration study has shown that the combination of hydralazine and isosorbide dinitrate significantly reduced mortality in heart failure patients unresponsive to digitalis and diuretics. Long-term therapy with hydralazine has been associated with the development of systemic lupus erythematosus, which presents as fatigue, malaise, low-grade fever, and joint aches and pains. Baseline and serial blood counts for antinuclear antibody titers should be performed; if systemic lupus erythematosus develops, discontinuation of the drug results in reversal of the symptoms over time.

31. The answer is E (I, II, and III).
Inocor (inamrinone), Dobutrex (dobutamine), and dopamine are inotropic agents. Inotropic agents have been used in the emergency treatment of patients with heart failure and in patients refractory to, or unable to take, digitalis. However, current guidelines provide a Class III recommendation, which states, "conditions for which there is evidence and/or general agreement that a procedure/therapy is not useful/effective and in some cases may be harmful." Additionally, current guidelines provide a Class IIb recommendation for the use of continuous intravenous infusion of a positive inotropic agent for palliation of heart failure symptoms, which states, "conditions for which there is conflicting evidence and/or a divergence of opinion about the usefulness/efficacy of performing the procedure/therapy and that the usefulness/efficacy is less well established by evidence/opinion."

32. The answer is A (I only).
Motrin (ibuprofen and other NSAIDs) have been reported to cause gastrointestinal erosions and ulcers. This patient could have a major problem because of a report of anemia.

33. The answer is E.
Similar to angiotensin-converting enzyme (ACE) inhibitors, β-adrenergic blockers work through actions of the endogenous neurohormonal system. Unlike ACE inhibitors, which work strictly by blocking the effects of the renin–angiotensin system, β-adrenergic blockers work by interfering with the sympathetic nervous system. This has prompted the use of three different types of β-adrenergic blockers: (1) those that are relatively selective towards β_1 receptors (i.e., metoprolol), (2) those that are selective to both β_1 and β_2 receptors (i.e., propranolol and bucindolol), and (3) those that are selective to β_1, β_2, and α_1 receptors (i.e., carvedilol). β-adrenergic blockers, similar to ACE inhibitors, have been shown to decrease the risk of death or hospitalization as well as improve the clinical status of heart failure patients. Current guidelines recommend the use of a β-adrenergic blocker in all patients with stable heart failure due to left ventricular dysfunction unless they have a contraindication to their use or are unable to tolerate their effects due to hypotension, bradycardia, bronchospasm, and the like.

34. The answer is C.
Atropine in therapeutic doses inhibits cholinergic impulses and increases the heart rate. When treatment is initiated in a patient with sinus bradycardia, initial small doses may actually stimulate cholin-

ergic receptors and therefore increase the degree of bradycardia. Constipation, dry mouth, decreased secretions, and pupillary dilation are all side effects associated with anticholinergic drugs. Rarely do single doses of atropine cause constipation.

35. The answer is A (I).
Quinidine is a class I_A antiarrhythmic agent, which has gastrointestinal intolerance as one of its side effects. Sustained-release products such as Quinaglute have been shown to reduce this effect by lowering the peak blood levels of quinidine. This reduction causes a more consistent, prolonged effect. Carvedilol (Coreg) is a β-adrenergic blocker and is indicated in the treatment of heart failure but is not available as a sustained-release product, nor is it indicated as an antiarrhythmic. Felodipine (Plendil) is not available as an extended-release product but it does have an extended half-life, which allows less frequent dosing in the treatment of hypertension. It is one of the second-generation calcium channel blocking agents and is not indicated as an antiarrhythmic agent.

36. The answer is D.
Inamrinone (Inocor) is a bipyridine agent that has both positive inotropic effects and vasodilating effects. It does offer an alternative to dopamine and dobutamine and is given as an IV infusion of 5 to 10 mcg/kg/min. Timolol (Blocadren) and atenolol (Tenormin) are β-adrenergic blockers, verapamil (Calan) is a calcium channel blocker, and disopyramide (Norpace) is a class I_A antiarrhythmic agent; all have negative inotropic activities. Their use could create a problem in a patient who requires inotropic support. β-adrenergic blockers are currently recommended as first-line agents in patients with stable heart failure unless they have a contraindication to their use or cannot tolerate their effects due to hypotension, bradycardia, bronchospasm, and the like.

37. The answer is D.
Lansoprazole (Prevacid) is a proton pump inhibitor used for the short-term treatment of refractory duodenal ulcer, severe erosive esophagitis, and poorly responsive gastroesophageal reflux disease. Cimetidine (Tagamet) and famotidine (Pepcid) are H_2-receptor antagonists that work by inhibiting the actions of histamine at the parietal cell receptor sites. Sucralfate (Carafate) is a nonabsorbable mucosal protectant that adheres to the base of ulcer craters. Octreotide (Sandostatin) is a long-acting synthetic octapeptide that works like somatostatin by inhibiting serotonin, gastrin, vasoactive intestinal polypeptide, insulin, glucagon, growth hormone, and other agents.

38. The answer is A.
Creatinine is formed during muscle metabolism, and creatinine clearance is the most common method for the measurement of glomerular filtration rate (GFR). When only the serum creatinine level and the patient's age, weight, and gender are known, creatinine clearance may be determined by the Cockroft and Gault equation.

39. The answer is E (I, II, and III).
Low doses of aspirin and other salicylates inhibit the tubular secretion of uric acid, which may result in uric acid accumulation and gout. Nicotinic acid competes with uric acid for excretion in the kidney tubule, resulting in greater retention of uric acid and the possibility of a gout attack. Cytotoxic drugs, by nature of their ability to increase nucleic acid turnover (uric acid is a byproduct of nucleic acid), cause an increase in uric acid and the potential for a gout attack.

40. The answer is C (I, II).
Oxymetazoline is a sympathomimetic vasoconstrictor; its effect lasts up to 12 hours. This agent is administered twice daily for up to 3 days.

41. The answer is A (I).
Ferrous salts are absorbed from the gastrointestinal tract better than ferric salts. Common ferrous salts include ferrous gluconate (Fergon), ferrous sulfate (Feosol), and ferrous fumarate (Femiron).

42. The answer is C.
The four clinical classes of diabetes mellitus are Type 1, Type 2, gestational diabetes mellitus, and secondary diabetes. Hyperglycemia is elevated blood sugar but is not identified as a "clinical class" of diabetes mellitus. Hyperglycemic nonketotic syndrome can occur in Type 2 diabetes where blood glu-

cose levels increase but without breakdown of fats because some insulin is present. Diabetic ketoacidosis may occur in patients with Type 1 diabetes. This results in hyperglycemia and breakdown of fats because of insulin insufficiency. Ketonemia (accumulation of ketone bodies in the blood) results from the breakdown of adipose tissue when there is insulin deficiency in Type 1 diabetes. Thiazide diuretics and Cushing's syndrome may result in hyperglycemia (secondary diabetes). There is no such thing as Type 3 diabetes.

43. The answer is C (I, II).
Items I and II in this question are diagnostic criteria for nonpregnant adults. To meet the diagnostic criteria for a oral glucose tolerance test, the plasma glucose level at the 2-hour mark must be at least 200 mg/dl. The pharmacist did not record any symptoms for Mr. Johnson. Because he received an oral glucose tolerance test, apparently his level was above 200 mg/dl.

44. The answer is E (I, II, and III).
Hemoglobin A1C is a useful long-term monitoring tool to measure glycemic control. It is usually tested at least once or twice per year in patients under good control and at least quarterly for therapy changes and those who are in poor control.

45. The answer is E (I, II, and III).
Glyburide is chemically classified as a sulfonylurea. These agents stimulate the pancreatic secretion of insulin (insulin secretagogue) and therefore result in lowered blood glucose (hypoglycemic agent).

46. The answer is C (I and II).
Diabeta, Micronase, and Glynase (not listed above) are trade names for glyburide. Glucotrol is glipizide, another sulfonylurea agent.

47. The answer is E (I, II, and III).
Glucovance is a trade name for the combination product (glyburide and metformin). These two individual drugs can be used successfully in combination to treat Type 2 diabetes patients. Metformin has several mechanisms of action, but it is generally recognized as an insulin sensitizer. Situations such as renal dysfunction, chronic or binge alcohol ingestion, etc., can increase the risk for the development of lactic acidosis.

48. The answer is A (I).
This agent is an α-glucosidase inhibitor in the intestine and acts by reducing the absorption of carbohydrates (complex carbohydrate absorption requires the action of α-glucosidase). Postprandial blood glucose levels are therefore lower. These agents have little effect on preprandial or fasting blood glucose levels. This agent has an entirely different mechanism of action from metformin.

49. The answer is A (I).
As noted in I, urine glucose does not give current information about what is happening with the patient's blood glucose level. Self-monitoring of blood glucose (SMBG) is indicated for all patients with diabetes. Mr. Johnson would need to do urine ketone monitoring only if he were to develop an acute illness (i.e., infection) or if he were trying to actively lose weight by calorie restriction. This would not be a method for routine glucose monitoring.

50. The answer is C (I, II).
Osteoarthritis, formerly known as degenerative joint disease, is the most common form of arthritis. There is little, if any, inflammation in the osteoarthritic joint.

51. The answer is C (I, II).
The product contains the antihistamine diphenhydramine. Diphenhydramine and doxylamine are the two FDA-approved OTC agents indicated for insomnia. Diphenhydramine may produce adverse central anticholinergic effects in the elderly, including confusion, disorientation, impaired short-term memory, and, at times, visual and tactile hallucinations. Because of its anticholinergic properties, diphenhydramine may cause restriction in the urinary outflow in a male patient with an enlarged prostate. It would not cause polyuria.

52. The answer is D (II, III).
Sonata (zaleplon) has a short terminal half-life (about 1 hour) and decreases sleep latency and at this dose would be more useful for individuals having difficulty falling asleep. The 5-mg dose is appropriate for a elderly man. It can be used for up to 4 to 5 hours before the individual has to get up due to its short half-life.

53. The answer is B.
Because there is little, if any, inflammation in the osteoarthritic joint, acetaminophen has been shown to be as efficacious as ibuprofen and naproxen in patients with mild to moderate osteoarthritic pain. It is considered by the American College of Rheumatology as first-line therapy for osteoarthritis of the hip or knee. It generally has fewer side effects than the NSAIDs, and usually it is used initially. Mr. Johnson was initially "prescribed" acetaminophen for this condition, which was the correct choice.

54. The answer is A.
The dose should be adequate to control the patient's pain. Hepatotoxicity, the main concern, can occur in patients taking greater than 4 g acetaminophen per day. Symptoms can include nausea, vomiting, abdominal pain, malaise, and diaphoresis.

55. The answer is E (I, II, and III).
Elderly patients and those with a history of peptic ulcer disease are at increased risk for gastrointestinal toxicity when taking NSAIDs. Tramadol is considered a good choice, after acetaminophen, in patients who cannot tolerate NSAID use. Tramadol is not a narcotic analgesic, but side effects such as nausea, constipation, and somnolence occur with both tramadol and opioids.

56. The answer is E (I, II, and III).
Robitussin Cold Multisymptom Cold & Flu Caplets contains acetaminophen, pseudoephedrine, guaifenesin, and dextromethorphan. Before recommending an OTC product for the treatment of the common cold, we need to know what symptoms the patient is experiencing and then target our therapy to those symptoms, most likely with a single-ingredient product. Since he is experiencing what he describes as a common cold and it is summertime, is it truly a common cold, or is he experiencing symptoms of seasonal allergic rhinitis? Pseudoephedrine administration may result in increasing Mr. Johnson's blood sugar, so this agent should be used cautiously (if at all) in patients with diabetes. This product does contain 250 mg acetaminophen, which may push Mr. Johnson over the 4 g maximum daily allotment of acetaminophen. Finally, this product contains sucrose, which could affect Mr. Johnson's blood sugar level. Sugar-free products should be substituted if the product was deemed appropriate in the first place.

57. The answer is A (I).
The insulin secretagogues (e.g., the sulfonylurea, glyburide) may not work to control blood sugar during the first 4 weeks of therapy (primary). This is likely due to the insufficient number of functioning β-cells in the pancreas. Secondary failure occurs when the drug controls hyperglycemia initially but fails to maintain the control. In most cases, this represents a progression of the diabetes rather than a "drug failure."

58. The answer is D.
The directions in item D indicate how to treat this form of seborrhea of the scalp in the newborn. This procedure will gently remove the accumulated scaly skin.

59. The answer is C.
It is generally believed that the absorptive characteristics of the skin in children under the age of 6 months are different from those of adults. The metabolic and excretory systems of these young children may not be able to handle the sunscreen agent that does get absorbed.

60. The answer is B.
Salicylic acid is a keratolytic agent and is considered safe and effective for the treatment of warts by the FDA. It is also used for the treatment of corns and calluses.

61. The answer is E.
Human papillomavirus is the cause of common warts. Herpes simplex virus Type I is responsible for cold sores, Type 2 for genital herpes. The Epstein-Barr virus is the usual cause of infectious mononucleosis. Coronavirus is one of the viruses responsible for the common cold. HIV is the human immunodeficiency virus.

62. The answer is C.
Appropriate treatment measures are listed in items A, B, D, and E. All bedrooms (where the concentration of pinworm eggs is likely to be the greatest) should be vacuumed instead of swept to remove the eggs.

63. The answer is A.
According to the recommendations of the JNC-7 (a multidisciplinary, national collaborative group), drug therapy is usually initiated with a thiazide diuretic in patients with Stage I hypertension not associated with any of the "compelling" indications. However, additional recommendations include alternative therapy with angiotensin-converting enzyme inhibitors, angiotensin II receptor blockers, β-adrenergic receptor blockers, or calcium channel blockers for patients who are unable to tolerate a thiazide diuretic or who do not respond appropriately to them. Spironolactone is a potassium-sparing diuretic that antagonizes aldosterone receptors within the distal convoluted tubule and has minor diuretic effects. Doxazosin is a peripherally acting α-adrenergic blocker that demonstrated potentially negative clinical effects in the recent ALLHAT study. Hydralazine is a vasodilator that directly dilates peripheral arteries to reduce blood pressure. Clonidine is a centrally acting antihypertensive that stimulates α2-adrenergic receptors to decrease sympathetic outflow to lower blood pressure. None of these agents is considered an alternative to thiazide diuretics as initial therapy for Stage I hypertension.

64. The answer is B (III).
The individual reviewing the orders identified that hydrochlorothiazide (HCTZ) is a sulfa derivative, and due to the nature of the previously documented allergy, specifically Stevens-Johnson syndrome (a type of erythema multiforme reaction) was able to inform the prescriber so that spironolactone, which is not a sulfa derivative (although it is considerably less potent than HCTZ), was prescribed. Previous studies have demonstrated the benefit of thiazide diuretics on mortality rates in hypertensive patients. However, additional considerations in the current patient should include the potential use of angiotensin-converting enzyme inhibitors, angiotensin II receptor blockers, β-adrenergic receptor blockers, and/or calcium channel blockers because this patient cannot take a thiazide diuretic.

65. The answer is C.
The development of ischemic heart disease involves the relationship between oxygen supplied to the heart and oxygen demanded by the heart. Similar to a balance, when these two parameters are equal, the heart is able to provide oxygen to the metabolizing tissues, which they need to maintain normal bodily functions. However, the inability for the supply of oxygen to increase as demands placed on the heart are increased can result in an acute coronary syndrome. Heart rate, cardiac contractility, fluid volume within the cardiac ventricles, and the wall tension within the cardiac ventricles directly reflect the oxygen demands placed on the heart. Coronary blood flow is a direct reflection of the degree of oxygen supplied to the heart. As oxygen supply is reduced, coronary blood flow is reduced (atherosclerosis, vasospasm); as oxygen demand is increased (increased heart rate, increased ventricular size, increased cardiac contractility), the balance between supply and demand is altered and can result in ischemic heart disease in predisposed patients.

66. The answer is E (I, II, and III).
"Acute ischemic (coronary) syndromes" is a term that has evolved as a way to describe a group of clinical symptoms representing acute myocardial ischemia. The clinical symptoms include acute myocardial infarction, which might include ST-segment elevation (STEMI) or ST segment depression (NSTEMI), it might include a Q wave or non-Q wave infarction, or it might be considered unstable angina. Current terminology has not included angina pectoris as one of the acute coronary syndromes.

67. The answer is D.
Theophylline serum levels are increased by conditions that decrease theophylline elimination. Smoking increases the rate of theophylline elimination by increasing the rate of metabolism, resulting in a reduced serum theophylline level. Pneumonia, ciprofloxacin, cor pulmonale, and heart failure decrease the rate of theophylline elimination, resulting in an increased serum theophylline level.

68. The answer is B (III).
Atenolol is a β-adrenergic blocking agent, which is referred to as a relatively cardioselective agent. However, no β-adrenergic blocking agent is entirely safe in an asthmatic patient such as Mr. Torres because it might induce a bronchospastic attack. Spironolactone, a potassium-sparing diuretic, and irbesartan, an angiotensin II receptor blocker, can be prescribed for asthmatic patients because they do not affect the respiratory system.

69. The answer is D.
All of the agents listed are calcium channel blockers and have been used successfully in the treatment of hypertension. However, within the calcium channel blockers, there are three different chemical groups; amlodipine, nifedipine, felodipine, and isradipine are referred to as dihydropyridine derivatives, which do not slow impulses within the atrioventricular (AV) node. Verapamil has been shown to effectively slow impulses within the AV node and has been used in the treatment of tachyarrhythmias, angina pectoris, and hypertension.

70. The answer is D (II, III).
All three of the agents are referred to collectively as HMG-CoA reductase inhibitors. Additional agents include lovastatin, fluvastatin, and atorvastatin. To date, several studies have shown that pravastatin and simvastatin can reduce the mortality rate from coronary artery disease when administered to patients with hypercholesterolemia. Cerivastatin was recently removed from the market due to consequences associated with its use, resulting in liver damage in select patients.

71. The answer is B (III).
Olmesartan is a member of a large class of agents referred to as angiotensin II type I receptor antagonists, which decrease the conversion of angiotensin I to angiotensin II. This results in a reduction in the release of aldosterone as well as a reduction in the powerful vasoconstrictor effects of angiotensin II. Centrally acting α-adrenergic agonists such as clonidine have been available for several years, and the identification of a purely cardiospecific β-adrenergic blocker has yet to occur. Several β-blockers have been shown to be relatively cardioselective, which results in greater β1 inhibition within the myocardium rather than β2 inhibition within the peripheral vascular system and pulmonary system. However, cardioselective properties are dose dependent, and to date no β-adrenergic blocker has been shown to possess strictly β1-inhibiting properties.

72. The answer is E (I, II, and III).
In most patients, the cause of Parkinson's disease is unknown (idiopathic); however, a small percentage of cases are secondary, and many of these cases are curable. Secondary parkinsonism may be caused by drugs, including dopamine antagonists (phenothiazine, butyrophenones such as haloperidol, reserpine), poisoning by chemicals such as carbon monoxide poisoning, heavy metals such as manganese or mercury, infectious diseases such as viral encephalitis and syphilis, as well as other causes, which include arteriosclerosis, degenerative diseases of the central nervous system, and various metabolic disorders.

73. The answer is B (III).
Diphenhydramine is an antihistaminic agent that has some mild anticholinergic effects and is used for symptomatic release of mild tremor. Amantadine is a dopaminergic agent. Trihexyphenidyl is an anticholinergic agent. Treatment of Parkinson's disease usually involves the use of antihistaminic drugs, anticholinergic agents, and dopaminergic agents. Due to its adverse reaction within the central nervous system, diphenhydramine should be used with caution in the elderly.

74. The answer is C.
Biperiden is an anticholinergic agent used in the treatment of Parkinson's disease; the daily dosage range is 2 to 8 mg. Benztropine, another anticholinergic agent, has a daily dosage range of 1 to 6 mg. Pramipexole, referred to as a non-ergot dopamine agent, has a daily dosage range of 1.5 to 4.5 mg. Tolcapone (300–600 mg/day) and entacapone (200–1600 mg/day) are referred to as catechol-O-methyltransferase (COMT) inhibitors.

75. The answer is C (I, II).
Entacapone, a catechol-O-methyltransferase (COMT) inhibitor, works by delaying the metabolism of levodopa and therefore prolonging its availability. It is therefore indicated as an adjunctive treatment to levodopa in patients who suffer from a "wearing off" effect.

76. The answer is A.
Caution is needed when introducing anticholinergics in this patient with narrow-angle glaucoma. Anticholinergic agents may aggravate certain other underlying conditions and therefore should also be used with caution in patients with obstructions of the gastrointestinal or genitourinary tracts or severe cardiac disease. Side effects usually include dry mouth, blurred vision, constipation, urinary retention, and tachycardia. Central nervous system side effects may include hallucinations, ataxia, mental slowing, confusion, and memory impairment.

77. The answer is E (I, II, and III).
Levodopa in capable of causing adverse drug reactions within the gastrointestinal (anorexia, nausea, vomiting, abdominal distress), cardiovascular (postural hypotension and tachycardia), and musculoskeletal (dystonia or choreiform muscle movement) systems. Additional organ systems with associated adverse reactions include the central nervous system (confusion, memory changes, depression, hallucinations, and psychosis) and the hematologic system (hemolytic anemia, leukopenia, and agranulocytosis).

78. The answer is B (III).
Anticholinergic agents should be given one drug at a time. Several agents are available for therapy, and they all appear to be equally effective. One of the principles of drug therapy is that if a patient does not respond to an agent in one class, try another class. The exception includes the use of dopamine agonists, bromocriptine, and pergolide; patients who do not respond to one of the agents may not respond to the other.

79. The answer is D.
Of the drugs listed (chlorphenoxamine, biperiden, mesoridazine, pergolide, and perphenazine), only pergolide is a dopaminergic agent. Available dopaminergic agents and their mechanisms include levodopa, which exogenously replenishes striatal dopamine; bromocriptine, which directly stimulates dopamine receptors; amantadine, which stimulates presynaptic dopamine release; pergolide, which directly stimulates dopamine receptors in the nigrostriatal system; selegiline, which selectively inhibits monoamine oxidase type B and selectively prevents the breakdown of dopamine in the brain; pramipexole and ropinirole, which are considered non-ergot dopamine agents; and tolcapone and entacapone, referred to as COMT inhibitors, which delay the breakdown of dopamine in the brain.

80. The answer is A.
Levodopa must be converted to dopamine, and this conversion must occur centrally, for therapeutic effect. Because dopamine does not readily cross the blood–brain barrier, it is important that only minimal amounts of levodopa be converted to dopamine peripherally. The enzyme for this metabolic reaction is dopa-decarboxylase, for which pyridoxine (vitamin B6) is a coenzyme. Exogenous pyridoxine can therefore increase the peripheral metabolism of levodopa, making less dopamine available centrally for the desired effect.

81. The answer is A (I).
Carbidopa inhibits the peripheral decarboxylation of levodopa to dopamine. Carbidopa does not cross the blood–brain barrier, therefore making more levodopa available for transport to the brain. This situation minimizes the risk of peripheral side effects and may lower the required dose of levodopa by approximately 75%.

82. The answer is B.
The "on–off" phenomenon refers to swings in drug response to levodopa or dopamine agonists. Loss of drug effectiveness is characteristic of "off" periods. Bromocriptine, a dopamine agonist, has been shown to be effective in patients who have responded poorly to levodopa or who have experienced a severe on–off phenomenon. It is often used as an adjunct to levodopa therapy. Pergolide is a similarly acting agent that has been shown to be 1000 times more potent than bromocriptine on a milligram basis.

83. The answer is B (III).
Significance is generally determined by statistics, using an analysis of variance. A probability of $P \leq 0.05$ indicates a statistically significant difference (i.e., one that is not due to chance alone). Thus, the high-fat breakfast treatment had a longer T_{max} and a lower C_{max}, indicating a delay in absorption. The slower rate of systemic drug absorption may have been caused by a delay in stomach emptying time due to the ingestion of fat.

84. The answer is D.
Mechlorethamine (Mustargen) is nitrogen mustard, which serves as an alkylating agent. Chlorambucil (Leukeran), busulfan (Myleran), and melphalan (Alkeran) are all considered water-soluble compounds, which alkylate (alkylating agents) DNA. Doxorubicin (Adriamycin) is an example of a tetracyclic amino sugar-linked antibiotic.

85. The answer is A.
Dospan is an erosion-core tablet that employs insoluble plastics, hydrophilic polymers, or fatty compounds to create a matrix device. The slowly dissolving tablet releases the majority of a dose after the primary dose is released from the tablet coating. OROS is an osmotic delivery system. The transdermal drug delivery system (TDDS) is designed to support the passage of drug substances from the skin surface. Pennkinetic is an ion-exchange resin. The hydrodynamically balanced drug delivery system (HBS) represents a hydrocolloid system.

86. The answer is C.
Moxifloxacin, levofloxacin, ciprofloxacin, and gatifloxacin are all quinolone derivatives. Clarithromycin is a macrolide antibiotic claimed to be slightly more active than erythromycin against select gram-positive bacteria.

87. The answer is E (I, II, and III).
Immunosuppressive agents are administered to prevent graft rejection after renal transplantation. Azathioprine interferes with DNA and RNA synthesis so that it may reduce cell-mediated and humoral immune responses. Basiliximab is a chimeric monoclonal antibody that binds to block the interleukin-2 receptor on the surface of activated T lymphocytes, thus preventing T-lymphocyte activation and preventing acute rejection. Cyclosporine inhibits T-cell activation in the early stage of immune response to foreign antigen such as a graft.

88. The answer is A (I).
Captopril represents the class of drugs referred to as angiotensin-converting enzyme (ACE) inhibitors, which have been shown to provide a beneficial effect when given in the post-myocardial infarction stage to reduce morbidity and mortality from the myocardial infarction and prevention of left ventricular dysfunction. The Survival and Ventricular Enlargement (SAVE) trial was the first major study to show the direct benefits of ACE inhibitors in post-myocardial infarction patients. In Ms. Cunningham, the order for captopril was written approximately 3 days after the patient's heart attack and the dose was slowly titrated upward to prevent untoward hypotensive effects of the drug. Recent studies show that ACE inhibitors have a beneficial effect in certain patient populations (diabetes mellitus) in the prevention of renal nephropathy, but Ms. Cunningham is not receiving captopril for this reason. Additionally, ACE inhibitors do have a blood pressure-lowering effect, and although Ms. Cunningham may have received the drug for high blood pressure, she most likely received the drug for prevention of left ventricular dysfunction after the acute myocardial infarction.

89. The answer is B.
Levothyroxine has become the agent of choice for the treatment of hypothyroidism by virtue of its predictable results and the absence of triiodothyronine (T_3)-induced side effects. The usual adult maintenance dose of levothyroxine is 100 to 200 µg/day.

90. The answer is C (I, II).
The patient is experiencing symptoms of hyperthyroidism, which may reflect an excessive levothyroxine dose. In addition, amiodarone has been shown to produce both hypo- and hyperthyroid states.

91. The answer is E.
Amiodarone has an extremely long half-life—up to 50 days. The therapeutic effect of amiodarone may be delayed for weeks after oral therapy begins, and adverse reactions may persist up to 4 months after therapy ends.

92. The answer is C (I, II).
Propranolol is a β-adrenergic blocking agent that helps to reduce some peripheral manifestations of hyperthyroidism (e.g., tachycardia, sweating, tremor). In addition to providing symptomatic relief, propranolol inhibits the peripheral conversion of thyroxine (T_4) to triiodothyronine (T_3).

93. The answer is D (II, III).
Numerous large, multisite studies have been conducted comparing the various thrombolytic agents used in the management of acute myocardial infarction. The Global Utilization of Strategies to Open Occluded Arteries (GUSTO) study was developed to compare the impact of an accelerated administration of t-PA (over 1.5 hours) compared with traditional streptokinase or a combination of streptokinase and t-PA. The literature reveals that the ability to administer t-PA quickly in a shortened period of time ("front-loaded" regimen) is followed by a decrease in the time necessary for an occluded coronary artery to open or reperfuse, and results in a reduction in mortality. Cost issues continue to be significant in the selection of an ideal thrombolytic agent. t-PA is significantly more expensive than streptokinase on an ingredient-to-ingredient comparison. Recent economic evaluations have been conducted in which global costs of patient care, length of hospital stay, and so on have demonstrated an added benefit of t-PA.

94. The answer is B (III).
β-adrenergic blockers have been shown to be effective in the acute management of myocardial infarction patients in the prevention of sudden cardiac death due to acute myocardial infarction. They are also indicated in the treatment of angina pectoris, hypertension, and tachyarrhythmias, along with numerous other drug-specific indications. However, the acute administration of a β-blocker (primarily atenolol and metoprolol) has become an important part of the treatment of acute myocardial infarction. Whichever agent is used, usually a series of IV administrations of the drug are given over a short period of time, and then the patient is converted to oral medication daily thereafter. The parameters that need to be evaluated in these patients include blood pressure (if too low, the patient cannot receive a β-blocker), heart rate (if too low, the patient cannot receive a β-blocker), and pulmonary/left ventricular function (patients with signs of heart failure may not be candidates for β-blocker therapy).

95. The answer is B (III).
The patient has a reported allergy history that is consistent with quinidine-induced cinchonism, a consequence of an elevated quinidine serum level. If left unaltered, it can progress to delirium and psychosis, but the therapy of choice is to reduce the dose of quinidine, with a resultant decrease in the quinidine serum level and a potential reduction in symptoms. Aluminum hydroxide gel has been shown effective in the prevention of diarrhea, which has been reported to occur in up to 30% of patients receiving quinidine. Desensitization of patients to quinidine by administering very small doses of quinidine over an accelerated period of time has not become a standard of practice for patients with reported allergies to quinidine. Most patients can be successfully maintained on an alternative antiarrhythmic agent.

96. The answer is C (I, II).
There are numerous causes for acute renal failure (ARF), which is a sudden, potentially reversible interruption of kidney function, resulting in the retention of nitrogenous waste products in body fluids. ARF is classified according to its cause. In prerenal ARF, impaired renal perfusion occurs due to dehydration, hemorrhage, vomiting, urinary losses from excessive diuresis, decreased cardiac output due to heart failure, or severe hypotension. Intrarenal ARF reflects structural kidney damage due to nephrotoxins such as aminoglycosides, severe hypotension, malignant hypertension, and radiation. Postrenal ARF occurs due to obstruction of urine flow along the urinary tract as a result of uric acid crystals, thrombi, bladder obstruction, etc. Mr. Rones has a history of heart failure and hypertension, which are both capable of causing ARF. Hyperkalemia does not cause ARF, but rather ARF is associated with hyperkalemia, which might be considered a medical emergency.

97. The answer is E.
Mr. Rones has reported allergies to sulfonamides and penicillin, so he should not be given any of the medications. Penicillin V potassium (V-Cillin-K) is a penicillin. Although the pharmacist may not know the exact nature of the reported allergy, a conversation with the physician would answer the question of whether an allergy exists. Trimethoprim-sulfamethoxazole (Bactrim, Septra) and hydrochlorothiazide are both sulfonamide derivatives; again, the pharmacist may not know the exact nature of the reported allergy, but a follow-up conversation with the physician should take place before filling either of these prescriptions for the patient.

98. The answer is E (I, II, and III).
Slow-K is a potassium supplement used to prevent hypokalemia. However, Mr. Rones is diagnosed as having hyperkalemia, probably secondary to acute renal failure, and he should not receive the pre-

scription. Additionally, moexipril, an angiotensin-converting enzyme inhibitor, is contraindicated in hyperkalemia due to its potassium-retaining properties. Sudafed (pseudoephedrine HCl) is an indirect-acting sympathomimetic that stimulates receptors, resulting in the release of adrenergic amines; it must be used with great caution in this hypertensive patient. The pharmacist should contact the physician before dispensing either of these prescriptions to determine whether the physician does indeed want to use them.

99. The answer is A (I).
Mr. Rones has heart failure as a "compelling" indication, which would suggest the use of diuretics, angiotensin-converting enzyme inhibitors (ramipril), angiotensin II receptor blockers (candesartan), β-adrenergic blockers (atenolol), or an aldosterone antagonist such as spironolactone. However, due to the presence of hyperkalemia in this patient, ramipril and candesartan should be avoided if possible.

100. The answer is C.
Situations that favor the development of hypokalemia (use of non–potassium-sparing diuretics, failure to administer potassium supplements, administration of agents that decrease serum potassium—Kayexalate, or sodium polystyrene sulfonate) have been reported to be able to cause digoxin toxicity because of the development of hypokalemia. Phenytoin and lidocaine have both been shown to be effective in the treatment of digoxin toxicity–induced arrhythmias. Digoxin is primarily eliminated in the active form via the kidney, but when renal function decreases, as in advancing age, the elimination of the drug is decreased. Monitoring for renal function can help prevent the development of digoxin toxicity.

101. The answer is D (II and III).
Felodipine and isradipine are referred to as second-generation dihydropyridine derivatives, similar in action to nifedipine, which make up the class of calcium channel blockers. Ramipril and enalapril are two examples from the class of angiotensin-converting enzyme (ACE) inhibitors. Losartan is an example of the class of drugs referred to as angiotensin II receptor antagonists, and atenolol, carvedilol, and propranolol are examples of the β-adrenergic receptor antagonist class of drugs.

102. The answer is E.
Patients such as Mr. Rones who have renal failure lose their ability to eliminate potassium from the kidney, and consequently elevations in serum potassium should be expected. Situations that favor the reabsorption of potassium by the kidney (administration of potassium supplements, use of potassium-sparing diuretics [spironolactone, ACE inhibitors, angiotensin 2 receptor blockers]) should be avoided. However, situations that promote the removal of potassium by the body (dialysis), potassium-removing resin (sodium polystyrene sulfonate), pharmacologic antagonists (calcium chloride or gluconate), or shift potassium intracellularly (regular insulin with dextrose) are used to treat hyperkalemia.

103. The answer is E (I, II, and III).
Verapamil (Isoptin) and atenolol (Tenormin) are representatives of the calcium channel blocker and β-adrenergic blocker groups and, as such, possess negative inotropic and negative chronotropic effects. Patients should be advised to check their heart rates and report any symptoms that represent side effects from the negative inotropic effects of these agents. This helps to prevent the development of signs of heart failure.

104. The answer is B.
The American Hospital Formulary Service (AHFS) provides yearly updates on available products as well as dosage forms, indications, adverse drug reactions, and other information on products available in the United States. In addition, throughout the year, AHFS publishes supplements that provide updates on newly released agents. Newly released agents are not immediately described in the AHFS, but they do appear in supplements shortly after their release. Of the resources listed, AHFS offers the greatest benefit. Most recently, AHFS has become available in the personal desk assistant (PDA) format, and updates are provided regularly. *Merck Index, Trissel's, Hansten's,* and *Physicians' Desk Reference (PDR)* do not provide updates throughout the year, so they would not provide much help on a newly released product. *Trissel's* focuses on injectable drug products, *Hansten's* on drug interactions.

105. The answer is D.
Digoxin (Lanoxin) had previously been widely considered the mainstay in the treatment of heart failure. However, its use, particularly in chronic heart failure, has become somewhat controversial, and

recent guidelines have encouraged its use in the short-term management of acute symptoms. Current recommendations favor the use of angiotensin-converting enzyme (ACE) inhibitors as primary therapy, with the addition of a diuretic if accompanied by shortness of breath. Digoxin does possess two pharmacologic effects that reflect its concentration within the body. With lower total body stores (8–12 μg/kg), digoxin exerts a positive inotropic effect on the myocardium: an increase in cardiac output and renal blood flow and a decrease in cardiac filling pressure, venous and capillary pressures, heart size, and fluid volume. With higher total body stores (15–18 μg/kg), digoxin produces negative chronotropic effects—a reduction in electrical impulse conduction from the sinoatrial node throughout the atria into the atrioventricular node.

106. The answer is E.
It takes approximately 4 to 5 half-lives, with no loading doses given, for a patient to reach steady-state serum digoxin concentrations. For an anephric patient, who has a terminal half-life of 3.5 to 4.5 days, 15 to 20 days would be required to reach a steady state. If the patient is in acute heart failure, the treatment of choice is rapid loading of enough digoxin to obtain total body stores of 8 to 12 μg/kg over a 12-hour period, followed by daily maintenance doses. The patient who has normal renal function needs approximately 6 to 8 days of daily maintenance doses to reach steady state, if loading doses are not given.

107. The answer is E.
Acebutolol (Sectral) is a long-acting, relatively cardioselective agent that may be beneficial in patients who have lung disease and need to receive fewer doses per day to increase compliance. All β-adrenergic blockers have the potential to cause bronchospasm in patients with suspected lung disease, but the cardioselective agents may provide benefit in lower doses. Timolol (Blocadren) lacks cardioselectivity but is longer-acting. Esmolol (Brevibloc) is available only in intravenous form and has a very short half-life of approximately 9 minutes. Nadolol (Corgard) is a long-acting agent without cardioselective properties. Propranolol (Inderal LA) would offer no more cardioselective properties than those of Inderal.

108. The answer is A (I).
Isosorbide dinitrate (Isordil) and other nitrates have been shown to reduce pulmonary congestion and increase cardiac output by reducing preload and perhaps afterload. Nitrates generally cause venous dilation, with a resultant increase in venous pooling and a reduction in venous return and preload. The combination of nitrates with hydralazine (arteriole dilator) has been shown to reduce morbidity and mortality in patients with heart failure. However, the combination should not be used as initial therapy over angiotensin-converting enzyme (ACE) inhibitors, but should be considered in patients who are intolerant of ACE inhibitors. Dopamine and dobutamine are inotropic agents, and current guidelines provide a Class III recommendation ("conditions for which there is evidence and/or general agreement that a procedure/therapy is not useful/effective and in some cases may be harmful"). Additionally, current guidelines provide a Class IIb recommendation for the use of continuous intravenous infusion of a positive inotropic agent for palliation of heart failure symptoms ("conditions for which there is conflicting evidence and/or a divergence of opinion about the usefulness/efficacy of performing the procedure/therapy and that the usefulness/efficacy is less well established by evidence/opinion").

109. The answer is B.
Martindale's Extra Pharmacopoeia is an international publication that may help identify products from markets outside the United States. *Facts and Comparisons, Identidex,* the *Physicians' Desk Reference (PDR),* and *Drug Information 1990* focus on products available in the United States.

110. The answer is A.
Peritoneal dialysis is not practical for drugs that are highly bound to plasma or tissue proteins, are nonpolar or lipid-soluble, or have a large volume of distribution. Drugs that are polar and have a small apparent volume of distribution tend to have a larger concentration in plasma and highly perfused tissues. These polar drugs are more easily dialyzed in the case of drug intoxication.

111. The answer is E (I, II, and III).
An important potential problem with the use of herbal medications is the inability to retrieve up-to-date information on many herbal substances currently available through various vendors. Previously, the FDA Center for Food Safety and Applied Nutrition had published the Special Nutritional Adverse Event

Monitoring System website for dietary supplements. Unfortunately, the website had not been updated since 1999 and currently is no longer available. Prior to its removal, an extensive list had been developed of supplements considered unsafe by the FDA. All of the substances listed have been considered unsafe by the FDA due to the damage reported on various organ systems.

112. The answer is B.
Iron is available in different oral forms as ferrous gluconate, ferrous sulfate, and ferrous fumarate. Each form has a different iron content. Ferrous gluconate contains 12% elemental iron, ferrous sulfate 20%, and ferrous fumarate 33%.

113. The answer is C.
In extemporaneous compounding, various methods may be used to reduce the particle size of a drug, including levigation, pulverization by intervention, spatulation, or trituration. Geometric dilution is a method of mixing a small amount of a drug with a large amount of powder in a geometric progression so that the final powder mixture is homogeneous. Pulverization by intervention uses the addition of non-solvent.

114. The answer is E.
The total dose is 2.5 mg/kg/hr $\times$80 kg $\times$6 hr = 1200 mg. At a strength of 5 mg/ml, each 50-ml vial contains 250 mg. The number of vials needed for this patient can be calculated by dividing the total dose (1200 mg) by the amount of antibiotic per vial (250 mg) = 4.8 vials (5 vials).

115. The answer is B.
For most drugs with poor aqueous solubility, the dissolution rate (the rate at which the drug is solubilized) is the rate-limiting step for systemic drug absorption. Disintegration is the fragmentation of a solid dosage form into smaller pieces.

116. The answer is A (I).
Amprenavir, indinavir, and nelfinavir are referred to as protease inhibitors and are used in the treatment of human immunodeficiency virus (HIV) infection in combination with other groups of antiretroviral agents. Ritonavir and saquinavir are additional agents in this group of drugs. Zalcitabine, lamivudine, and stavudine are referred to as nucleoside reverse transcriptase inhibitors and are used in combination with protease inhibitors in the treatment of HIV. Delavirdine, efavirenz, and nevirapine are referred to as non-nucleoside reverse transcriptase inhibitors and are used in the treatment of HIV as well.

117. The answer is A (I).
The rate of dissolution of a weak acid drug is directly influenced by the surface area of the solid particles, the water-in-oil partition coefficient, and the concentration gradient between the drug concentrations in the stagnant layer and the bulk phase of the solvent. An increase in the pH of the medium will make the medium more alkaline, and the weak acid will convert to the ionized species, becoming more water-soluble. Increasing the particle size decreases the effective surface area of the solid drug. Increasing the viscosity of the medium slows the diffusion of drug molecules into the solvent.

118. The answer is A.
While the mechanism of action for lithium remains virtually unknown, this agent remains the therapy of choice for the treatment and prophylaxis of mania. Membrane stabilization, inhibition of norepinephrine release, accelerated norepinephrine metabolism, increased presynaptic reuptake of norepinephrine and serotonin, and decreased receptor sensitivity appear to be therapeutic properties of lithium.

119. The answer is D.
Equivalent weight (Li_2CO_3) = molecular weight/valence = 73.89/2 = 36.945.
mEq = drug (mg)/equivalent weight (mg) = 300/36.945 = 8.12 mEq

120. The answer is E (I, II, and III).
Lithium therapy is monitored effectively by periodic determinations of serum lithium levels. Therapeutic serum level ranges are: acute mania, initial therapy: 0.8 to 1.5 mEq/L; maintenance therapy: 0.6 to 1.2 mEq/L. A variety of factors can affect serum lithium levels; important among these are the time interval between the last dose and the taking of the blood sample, and concomitant drug therapy (e.g.,

thiazide diuretics may increase serum lithium levels; osmotic diuretics may lower them). If the patient were acutely manic on admission, it might indicate that he was not taking his lithium medication as prescribed.

121. The answer is A (I).
The minimum, or trough, plasma drug concentration is the most consistent of the three; it is always lowest just before the administration of the next dose. The best time to monitor serum lithium levels is 12 hours after the last dose—that is, just before the first dose of the day. The exact times for the peak drug concentration and the average drug concentration are uncertain for any individual patient. The drawing of a plasma sample to obtain a "peak" plasma level uses an approximate time for maximum absorption of the drug. The average plasma drug concentration cannot be obtained directly but is approximated by dividing the area under the curve (AUC) dosing interval by the time (T) of the dosage interval.

122. The answer is B.
Before any other measures are taken, a repeat lithium level should be obtained to assess the patient's situation. Adverse effects of lithium are usually related to the serum lithium level. Gastrointestinal distress, polyuria and polydipsia, fine hand tremor, and muscle weakness are symptoms usually associated with lithium serum concentrations below 1.5 mEq/L. Other symptoms, such as persistent gastrointestinal distress, coarse hand tremor, hyperirritability, slurred speech, confusion, and somnolence, may be warning signs of toxicity and are evident with serum levels between 1.5 and 2.5 mEq/L. Severe lithium toxicity usually occurs when levels exceed 3.0 mEq/L; levels this high may be life-threatening.

123. The answer is D.
Lithium is eliminated renally by glomerular filtration and competes with sodium for reabsorption in the renal tubules. Thiazide diuretics interfere with sodium reabsorption and therefore may favor lithium reabsorption, leading to elevated lithium levels.

124. The answer is B (III).
Paroxetine, sertraline, and fluoxetine represent three agents making up the group of agents referred to as selective serotonin reuptake inhibitors (SSRIs). Amitriptyline, doxepin, and protriptyline represent examples of tricyclic antidepressants. Amoxapine is a debenzoxazepine, which is a primary blocker of postsynaptic reuptake of norepinephrine. Trazodone is a triazolopyridine derivative that causes inhibition of serotonin reuptake as well as blocking serotonin and α-adrenergic receptors. Bupropion is a monocyclic antidepressant and a dopamine reuptake inhibitor but has no significant effect on norepinephrine or serotonin receptors.

125. The answer is D.
Tricyclic antidepressants appear to lower the seizure threshold; therefore, caution must be exercised when using these preparations in patients with a history of seizures. The incidence of seizures remains low and is usually associated with high doses of these agents.

126. The answer is A.
When initiating SSRI therapy, it is important to start at the lowest dose possible and titrate up. A titration schedule will help minimize side effects while reaching therapeutic serum drug concentrations.

127. The answer is D.
Of the agents listed, paroxetine (Paxil) has the highest incidence of adverse sexual side effects. These effects include a decrease in libido (6–14% of males and 1–9% of females), orgasm dysfunction (occurring in up to 10% of patients), impotence (2–8%), and delayed ejaculation (13–28%). Priapism, although rare, has also been reported with all of the SSRIs.

128. The answer is C.
Load dose: 200 mg/m^2 ×0.89 m^2 = 178 mg

129. The answer is D.
Furosemide (Lasix) is a loop diuretic that acts principally at the ascending limb of the loop of Henle, where it inhibits the cotransport of sodium and chloride from the luminal filtrate. Loop diuretics increase the excretion of water, sodium, and chloride.

130. The answer is C (I, II).
Topical OTC nasal decongestants are sympathomimetic amines and include, among others, phenyle-phrine (e.g., Neo-Synephrine) and xylometazoline (e.g., Otrivin). Pseudoephedrine is an oral decon-gestant and is not available as a topical nasal decongestant.

131. The answer is C (I, II).
JNC-7 recommendations include thiazide-type diuretics (chlorothiazide [Diuril]), either alone or in combination with one other agent (e.g., angiotensin-converting enzyme inhibitor, angiotensin receptor blocker, β-blocker, or calcium channel blocker), for first-line treatment of Stage 1 hypertension, if there are no indications for another type of drug. Tenormin (atenolol), a β-blocker, would therefore be con-sidered as a first-line agent. Catapres (clonidine) is an α_2-adrenergic agonist and is not part of this first-line list.

132. The answer is E (I, II, and III).
Tardive dyskinesia is characterized by a mixture of orofacial dyskinesia, tics, chorea, and athetosis. Symptoms usually appear while patients are receiving an antipsychotic; however, symptoms may ap-pear or worsen during periods of antipsychotic dose reduction or discontinuation. Therefore, a short drug holiday may reveal symptoms, allowing early detection. Recommendations for avoiding the on-set of tardive dyskinesia include using antipsychotic agents only when clearly indicated, keeping the daily dose as low as possible, and monitoring patients closely for symptoms of tardive dyskinesia. Also, chronic use of anticholinergic agents is not recommended because these agents may increase the risk of tardive dyskinesia.

133. The answer is A (I).
Parnate (tranylcypromine) is a monoamine oxidase (MAO) inhibitor. Serious adverse drug reactions have been reported in patients receiving MAO inhibitors with opioid drugs. These serious interactions (hypotension, hyperpyrexia, coma) have occurred in patients receiving MAO inhibitors with meperi-dine (Demerol) but have not been reported to occur with morphine. Meperidine should be considered contraindicated in patients receiving MAO inhibitors. NSAIDs, a group that includes ketorolac, do not produce adverse interactions with MAO inhibitors. If a narcotic is necessary, morphine may be used cautiously, although waiting 14 days between the onset of morphine therapy and the discontinuation of MAO inhibitor therapy would be judicious.

134. The answer is D.
Ondansetron (Zofran) was the first in a new class of agents that are selective 5-HT$_3$-receptor antago-nists, blocking serotonin both peripherally on vagal nerve terminals and centrally at the chemorecep-tor trigger zone for chemotherapy-induced and special postoperative cases of nausea and vomiting. Bupropion (Zyban) is available for use as an aid in smoking cessation. Sertraline (Zoloft) is a selective inhibitor of serotonin reuptake and an agent prescribed for the treatment of depression. Linezolid (Zyvox) is used in the treatment of resistant gram-positive bacterial infections such as vancomycin-resistant enterococcus. Simvastatin (Zocor) is an HMG coenzyme A reductase inhibitor used in the treatment of hypercholesterolemia.

135. The answer is A.
Aripiprazole (Abilify) is an atypical antipsychotic approved for the treatment of schizophrenia. Rabeprazole (Aciphex) is a proton pump inhibitor commonly used for gastroesophageal reflux disease and peptic ulcer disease. Butoconazole is an antifungal approved for use in the treatment of vulvo-vaginal candidiasis. Clotrimazole is an antifungal agent used in the treatment of susceptible fungal in-fections.

136. The answer is B.
Vitamin D increases the absorption of calcium. Citracal is a brand name for calcium citrate. Ascorbic acid (vitamin C), vitamin E, and pantothenic acid are other vitamins.

137. The answer is C.
Bentoquatam (Ivy-Block) is an organoclay that should be applied at least 15 minutes prior to poison ivy plant exposure and then every 4 hours for continued protection. Because the oleoresin (urushiol) can rapidly penetrate the skin, it should be washed off soon after exposure (within 10 minutes is ideal). Ob-

viously, learning how to identify the poison ivy plant and avoiding it would be the best way of preventing the dermatitis.

138. The answer is B (III).
Clarithromycin is classified as a macrolide antibiotic. Cefaclor is a cephalosporin antibiotic. Celebrex is a COX-2 NSAID.

139. The answer is B.
Omeprazole (Prilosec) is an inactive drug that becomes active at the parietal cells in the gastrointestinal tract. It has an antisecretory effect and inhibits gastric acid secretion by blocking the proton pump within cells in the gastrointestinal tract. The drug is formulated as enteric-coated granules that are pH sensitive and release the drug at a pH above 6.0. The granules also may be removed from the exterior capsule and administered, but if the granules are crushed, the enteric coating is destroyed.

140. The answer is A (I only).
Enbrel (etanercept) is a disease-modifying antirheumatic drug (DMARD) used to delay the progression of the disease. It requires subcutaneous administration and can be given either by a health care provider or ideally by the patient. Celecoxib and rofecoxib are two agents that represent a newer class of drugs referred to as cyclooxygenase-2 (COX-2) receptor inhibitors. Currently, they are indicated in the treatment of rheumatoid arthritis or osteoarthritis, similar to previous NSAIDs (COX-1-2 inhibitors), to manage the symptoms associated with the diseases. Current literature suggests that they may offer a benefit over traditional NSAIDs by reducing the gastrointestinal consequences associated with the traditional agents.

141. The answer is B (III only).
Hydroxychloroquine (Plaquenil) is a disease-modifying antirheumatic drug (DMARD); its therapeutic benefit may take up to 6 months to develop. Hydroxychloroquine is given in dosages of 400 mg/day and has been associated with severe and sometimes irreversible adverse effects on the eyes, skin, central nervous system, and bone marrow. Because the drug may have severe effects on the eyes, an ophthalmologist should check visual acuity every 3 to 6 months, with therapy being discontinued at the first signs of retinal toxicity.

142. The answer is A.
Plavix (clopidogrel bisulfate) is an antiplatelet drug indicated for the reduction of atherosclerotic events (myocardial infarction, stroke, and vascular death) in patients with atherosclerosis documented by recent stroke, recent myocardial infarction, or established peripheral arterial disease. Auranofin (Ridaura), methotrexate (Rheumatrex), penicillamine (Depen), and gold sodium thiomalate (Myochrysine) are collectively referred to as disease-modifying antirheumatic drugs (DMARDs). Like hydroxychloroquine (Plaquenil), they are added to first-line therapy to slow or delay progression of the disabling symptoms and effects of rheumatoid arthritis.

143. The answer is E (I, II, and III).
Celebrex (celecoxib) represents a class of NSAIDs referred to as COX-2 receptor inhibitors. Currently, they are indicated in the treatment of rheumatoid arthritis or osteoarthritis, similar to previous NSAIDs (COX-1 inhibitors), to manage the symptoms associated with these diseases. Current literature suggests that they might offer a benefit over traditional NSAIDs by reducing the gastrointestinal consequences associated with use of these agents. Naproxen (Naprosyn) is an NSAID that is also used in the treatment of rheumatoid arthritis. Relafen (nabumetone), also an NSAID agent, is believed to have a greater specificity for the COX-2 receptor than the COX-1 receptor; it has also been used in the symptomatic control of rheumatoid arthritis. Each agent could be a suitable alternative for ibuprofen, and celecoxib in particular might reduce the gastrointestinal side effects associated with the other NSAIDs.

144. The answer is E.
Adverse drug reactions that can be seen in the use of hydroxychloroquine include visual changes (as noted in question 141), agranulocytosis, and hemolytic anemia.

145. The answer is B (III).
Naprosyn (naproxen) is the only correct match. The generic name for Vioxx is rofecoxib; the generic name for Lodine is etodolac.

146. The answer is D (II, III).
Michaelis-Menten kinetics describes nonlinear pharmacokinetics in which a drug shifts from first-order to zero-order kinetics at higher doses when an enzyme system becomes saturated. This process also is known as capacity-limited, or saturation, pharmacokinetics.

147. The answer is B (III).
A well-known side effect of aspirin products is gastrointestinal bleeding due to the direct effects of aspirin on the gastrointestinal tract, as well as the systemic effect of aspirin on prostaglandin synthesis. Ms. Szymuniak's gastrointestinal bleeding has resulted in an anemia that necessitates the initiation of therapy with iron. The patient was given prescriptions also for vitamin B12 and folic acid. Folic acid might be justified, but not because of the gastrointestinal bleeding from the aspirin. There is hyperutilization of folic acid when the rate of cellular division is increased, as in chronic inflammatory diseases such as rheumatoid arthritis. Vitamin B12 supplementation would not be justified unless another type of anemia (pernicious anemia) was present. Later, the patient was given a prescription for Tagamet as treatment for the speculated ulcer, which developed from aspirin therapy. Finally, on 2/4, Cytotec and Maalox were added to prevent further damaging effects associated with aspirin therapy. The patient was finally switched to Motrin because she was unable to tolerate aspirin, even in the enteric-coated form.

148. The answer is C (I and II).
According to the guidelines established by the American College of Rheumatology, patients are diagnosed as having rheumatoid arthritis if they have satisfied at least four of the following seven criteria, with the first four continuing for at least 6 weeks: (1) morning stiffness, (2) arthritis in three or more joint areas, (3) arthritis of hand joints, (4) symmetric arthritis, (5) subcutaneous nodules (rheumatoid nodules), (6) abnormal serum rheumatoid factor, and (7) radiologic changes, with erosion or bone decalcification of involved joints.

149. The answer is E (I, II, and III).
Unfractionated heparin binds antithrombin III, which causes an accelerated inhibition of factor IIa (thrombin), factor Xa, and factor IXa.

150. The answer is C.
Tinea infections are superficial fungal dermatophyte infections of the skin. These infections are usually named based on the area of the skin involved: tinea cruris (groin), tinea capitis (head), tinea pedis (feet), tinea corporis (body), and tinea unguium (nails). Sally has tinea pedis.

151. The answer is D.
The antiseptic agent hexylresorcinol is not considered safe and effective for the treatment of tinea infections. The other four agents are all considered safe and effective for treating tinea pedis.

152. The answer is A.
Diphenhydramine and doxylamine are two ethanolamine antihistamines, generally considered the most sedating class of antihistamines. Brompheniramine, chlorpheniramine, dexbrompheniramine, and pheniramine are part of the alkylamine class of antihistamines, which are among the least sedating of the first-generation antihistamines. Thonzylamine, used very rarely today, is an ethylenediamine antihistamine; as a class, this is between the other two classes mentioned in terms of sedation effects. Loratadine is a second-generation nonsedating antihistamine that recently was moved to OTC status.

153. The answer is B.
One of the second-generation nonsedating antihistamines, loratadine (Claritin, others), is now available over the counter. This patient's specific symptoms are related to histamine effects, so an antihistamine is warranted. Given his occupation, we don't want to give this patient a sedating antihistamine such as diphenhydramine. Even though loratadine is considered a nonsedating antihistamine, a small percentage of patients experience somnolence (8%) and fatigue (4%). Mr. Conway should certainly see how this agent affects him before he attempts to drive. He does not have nasal congestion, so the decongestant (pseudoephedrine) is not warranted at this time.

154. The answer is A.
Nonsalicylate NSAIDs (ibuprofen, naproxen, and ketoprofen) are the most effective OTC agents for primary dysmenorrhea. Aspirin and acetaminophen are generally less effective. Ketoprofen is the correct answer here because it should be used OTC only in patients 16 years of age and older.

155. The answer is C (I and II).
Pyrethrins with piperonyl butoxide (synergized pyrethrins) and permethrin are the two safe and effective OTC agents to treat head lice. Patients should be warned to use these as directed as there is a growing trend of lice resistance to these products. Lindane is only available by prescription and has generally fallen into disfavor.

156. The answer is C.
Novolin is a trade name for human insulin that is a fixed-dose mixture of 70% NPH (intermediate action) and 30% Regular insulin (short action).

157. The answer is C (I, II).
The Tambocor and Coumadin prescriptions would be filled because they would have no adverse effect on Ms. Urmeister's allergy to aspirin. Ecotrin is a brand name for enteric-coated aspirin, which may be less irritating to the gastrointestinal tract but would still be contraindicated in this patient because she has an aspirin allergy. Aspirin has been shown to be effective as an antiplatelet agent in patients after a myocardial infarction, but as with any drug therapy, the benefits of use must be weighed against the associated risks.

158. The answer is E (I, II, and III).
Most antiarrhythmics fall into one of four classes, depending on their specific effects on the heart's electrical activity. Class I antiarrhythmic agents are divided into three groups based on their effects on depolarization rates and refractory period. Class IA drugs include quinidine, procainamide, and disopyramide; class IB drugs include lidocaine, tocainide, phenytoin, and mexiletine; class IC drugs include flecainide, propafenone, and moricizine.

159. The answer is D (II, III).
Sustained-release drug products allow for less frequent dosing, resulting in better patient compliance. Sustained-release forms also provide smoother plasma drug concentrations, with smaller fluctuations between peak and trough concentrations compared with immediate-release dosage forms of the drug. Procan SR is a sustained-release or extended-release dosage form of procainamide hydrochloride. Pronestyl capsules are an immediate-release form of the drug; Pronestyl SR is the sustained-release product.

160. The answer is E (I, II, and III).
Reteplase has been shown to be effective during the first several hours after a myocardial infarction to aid in the reperfusion of an infarcted coronary artery. Metoprolol, like other β-adrenergic receptor blocking agents administered shortly after an acute myocardial infarction, has been shown to be effective in reducing mortality and morbidity. In various studies, heparin has been shown to decrease the incidence of coronary reocclusion after the use of thrombolytic agents.

161. The answer is C (I, II).
Isosorbide dinitrate (Isordil) is used in both angina pectoris and heart failure. The development of angina pectoris centers around the balance between oxygen demand and oxygen supply to the myocardium. When the demand for oxygen exceeds the supply of oxygen, an angina attack occurs. Isosorbide dinitrate, like other nitrates, is a venous dilator resulting in reduced oxygen demand by the heart through a decrease in (venous return) preload. Isosorbide works in the heart failure patient by reducing venous return of blood to the heart, therefore, again, decreasing preload with a resultant decrease in fluid for the heart to pump. Clinical studies have demonstrated that the combination of isosorbide dinitrate with the arteriole dilator hydralazine has reduced mortality and morbidity in heart failure patients. Heart failure is a potential consequence of an acute myocardial infarction, and angina pectoris is a common underlying problem in many patients who have had a myocardial infarction. Both conditions are possible in Ms. Urmeister. Isosorbide dinitrate is not indicated in the acute treatment of hypertension.

162. The answer is C (I, II).
Isoproterenol is a sympathomimetic (β-adrenergic agonist) that increases oxygen demand by the heart through an increase in heart rate. Sympathomimetics, smoking, cold, and exercise all can increase oxygen demand, which may cause an acute angina attack or acute coronary syndrome in patients like Ms. Urmeister, who are at high risk. Acebutolol is a β-adrenergic receptor blocker that, like other β-blockers, reduces oxygen demand and is beneficial to patients with coronary artery disease.

163. The answer is A (I).
Bioavailability is a measurement of the rate and extent of systemic absorption of a drug, or the speed and amount that reaches the systemic circulation. For drug products to be bioequivalent, they must contain the same amount of active ingredient, must use the same route of administration, and must have the same bioavailability. The parameters Cmax, Tmax, and area under the curve (AUC) are used as a measurement of bioavailability of a drug. If these parameters are better than those for the parent product, the two products would not be considered equally bioavailable.

164. The answer is E.
Mexiletine (Mexitil) is an orally available drug that closely resembles lidocaine and is used to treat ventricular arrhythmias. As a class IB antiarrhythmic, like lidocaine, it can be considered a first-line agent in the treatment of ventricular tachycardia. Lidocaine must be administered parenterally, making it unsuitable in the ambulatory setting. Flecainide (Tambocor) and encainide (Enkaid) are class IC antiarrhythmics that are never indicated as first-line antiarrhythmics. Some physicians would argue that they should never be used; results of the Cardiac Arrhythmia Suppression Trial (CAST) study show that they can cause more harm than good. Encainide has already been removed from the market because of the major problems associated with its use. Dofetilide is a Class I antiarrhythmic that is indicated in the treatment of atrial fibrillation and atrial flutter. Distribution in the United States is through a restricted access process, and use requires inpatient treatment and close monitoring due to safety concerns.

165. The answer is B (III).
Quinidine (Quinidex) has been reported to cause diarrhea in as many as 30% of patients who receive the drug. Although loperamide (Imodium) may be helpful in stopping the diarrhea, patients often must discontinue the quinidine to stop it. Both aluminum hydroxide gel and polygalacturonate salt (Cardioquin) have been effective in combating quinidine-induced diarrhea.

166. The answer is B.
Morphine sulfate is a narcotic analgesic with venous pooling properties that reduce preload. Preload reduction decreases the oxygen demand placed on the heart. For this reason, along with its ability to alleviate pain and reduce anxiety (anxiety and pain also increase oxygen demand), morphine is frequently used in the myocardial infarction patient.

167. The answer is D (II, III).
The β-adrenergic blockers timolol (Blocadren) and atenolol (Tenormin) have been shown effective in preventing sudden death after myocardial infarction. Patients do need to be monitored closely for signs and symptoms of myocardial depression because these drugs may have negative inotropic and chronotropic effects. Procainamide (Procan SR) is a class IA antiarrhythmic agent used in the treatment of atrial and ventricular tachyarrhythmias.

168. The answer is C.
Nicoderm (nicotine) has been shown to be effective in helping patients stop smoking. Nitroglycerin patches are available in several brands (e.g., Nitro-Bid, Transderm-Nitro).

169. The answer is B.
Pseudoephedrine, a sympathomimetic amine, has CNS stimulating properties and is the most likely agent to cause sleep disruption. Metamucil (Psyllium) as a bulk laxative is not absorbed. Flonase (fluticasone) would be very unlikely. Benadryl (diphenhydramine) is one of the OTC agents used to treat insomnia would more likely cause drowsiness. CNS stimulation from regular doses of aspirin is highly unlikely.

170. The answer is E.
Middle ear infection (otitis media) and external ear infection (Swimmer's ear or otitis externa) require prescription antibiotics to treat. Water clogged ears can be treated with the OTC product containing isopropyl alcohol and anhydrous glycerin. Impacted cerumen can be treated with carbamide peroxide.

171. The answer is A.
Oxymetazoline has a duration of action of 12 hours and should be used no more than twice daily. The other topical nasal decongestants listed are administered every 6 hours (naphazoline), every 4 hours (phenylephrine, ephedrine), or every 2 hours (propylhexedrine).

172. The answer is B.
The SPF is the MED (minimal erythema dose) of sunscreen protected skin divided by the MED of unprotected skin. An SPF of 15 means that if the sunscreen was applied properly, the patient could stay out in the sun about 15 times longer to get a minimal sunburn as compared to when the skin is unprotected (i.e., no sunscreen application). 15 x 10 minutes = 150 minutes = 2 hours 30 minutes.

173. The answer is A.
If the patient misses a dose of Rogaine (Minoxidil), he should just continue with the next dose. One should not make up missed doses. The other items noted are appropriate counseling points to cover.

174. The answer is C.
Sulfur, salicylic acid, and sulfur + resorcinol are all considered safe and effective agents for the treatment of acne. Technically, benzoyl peroxide is currently classified as a Category III agent, meaning that more safety data is needed to determine that it does not have photocarcinogenic effects. Triclosan is an antibacterial agent with antigingivitis and antiplaque activity in the oral cavity with no proven efficacy against acne.

175. The answer is D.
Nonprescription treatment of acne is restricted to mild noninflammatory acne. It is clear that this young lady has more significant inflammatory acne. She has apparently had only a modest response to the OTC agents and she needs to be referred to a physician for additional prescription therapy.

176. The answer is D.
This agent is generally considered the nonprescription drug of choice for the treatment of acne. It does have a two-fold mechanism of action described in D above.

177. The answer is C.
If topical nasal decongestants are used for more often than 3–5 days, rhinitis medicamentosa (rebound congestion) may occur in the nasal passages. Thus, the patient ends up experiencing as a side effect what he sought to treat in the first place. For the common cold, a 3 to 5 day use of a topical nasal decongestant should be all that is needed.

178. The answer is D (II, III).
Tenuate Dospan is a controlled-release form of diethylpropion, a sympathomimetic agent. Many controlled-release drug products or modified dosage forms cannot be crushed because the integrity of the matrix would be destroyed and dangerous amounts of the active drug may be available for rapid absorption.

179. The answer is D (II, III).
First-order reactions are characterized by an exponential change in the drug amount or concentration with time, and these changes produce a straight line when plotted on a semilog graph. The half-life for a first-order reaction is a constant.

180. The answer is D (II and III).
Flumist is an inhaled influenza vaccine preparation approved for ages 5 to 49. The vaccine is viewed as unsafe in patients younger than 5 years due to concerns over increased rates of asthma within 42 days of vaccination. Safety and efficacy in patients 50 years and older have not been adequately assessed.

181. The answer is A.
Calcium is available for oral administration in a salt form of lactate, gluconate, phosphate, and carbonate; it is not available for oral administration in a salt form of chloride. Calcium chloride is available for IV injection. Dosage regimens should be individualized because of differences in calcium content.

182. The answer is C.
Osteonecrosis, hyperglycemia, fluid retention, and cataracts are long-term complications of therapy with steroids, including prednisone. Steroids generally increase the white blood cell count.

183. The answer is C.
Cidofovir suppresses cytomegalovirus replication by selective inhibition of DNA synthesis. It is not a protease inhibitor and is not indicated for treatment of HIV infection. Saquinavir (Invirase), ritonavir (Norvir), and indinavir (Crixivan) are protease inhibitors used to treat HIV infection.

184. The answer is A (I).
A pyrogen test is a fever test in rabbits or an in vitro test using the limulus (horseshoe crab). A positive test shows the presence of fever-producing substances (pyrogens) in a sterile product; these substances may be dead microorganisms or extraneous proteins.

185. The answer is A (I).
Increases in blood urea nitrogen (BUN) and serum creatinine generally indicate renal impairment. Levels of lactic dehydrogenase (LDG), aspartate aminotransferase (AST, formerly SGOT), and alanine aminotransferase (ALT, formerly SGPT) rise with liver dysfunction and indicate liver damage.

186. The answer is D.
Nausea and vomiting are common adverse reactions to chemotherapy; therefore, antiemetic therapy should be initiated before administration of chemotherapeutic drugs. Common antiemetic agents include ondansetron (Zofran), metoclopramide (Reglan), droperidol (Inapsine), and tetrahydrocannabinol (Marinol). Cimetidine (Tagamet) has no value as an antiemetic.

187. The answer is A.
Laboratory findings in acute renal failure include hyperuricemia, hyperkalemia, hypocalcemia, and metabolic acidosis. In acute renal failure, phosphate excretion decreases, causing hyperphosphatemia, not hypophosphatemia.

188. The answer is E.
Iodine is a trace element essential to the synthesis of thyroxine (T_4) and triiodothyronine (T_3). Iodine also is needed for physical and mental development and metabolism. Iodine deficiency can cause cretinism in children and infants.

189. The answer is B.
Omalizumab (Xolair) must be administered subcutaneously every 2 to 4 weeks. Injection site reactions occur in nearly half of patients.

Test II

Use the patient profile below to answer questions 1–8.

PATIENT RECORD—INSTITUTION/NURSING HOME

Patient Name: Thomas Anzalone
Address: 2098 West Central Ave
Age: 31   Height: 5'11"
Sex: M   Race: White   Weight: 185 lb
Allergies: Penicillin
Social History: 20 pack-year history

DIAGNOSIS
Primary   (1)   Acute schizophrenic episode
               (2)
Secondary   (1)
               (2)

LAB/DIAGNOSTIC TESTS

	Date	Test		Date	Test
(1)	8/14	Blood pressure 130/74	(5)		
(2)	8/14	Na 140; K 4; Cl 95;	(6)		
(3)		CO_2 25; BUN 11; Cr 1.0	(7)		
(4)	8/14	Hgb 12.5 g/dl; HCT 39%	(8)		

MEDICATION ORDERS Including Parenteral Solutions

	Date	Comments	Route	Sig
(1)	8/14	Haloperidol 5 mg	IM	stat
(2)	8/14	Haloperidol 5 to 10 mg	IM	q 4 h prn agitation
(3)	8/17	Risperidone	PO	2 mg bid

ADDITIONAL ORDERS

	Date	Comments
(1)	8/14	Admit to security ward
(2)	8/14	May restrain
(3)	8/17	D/C Haloperidol

DIETARY CONSIDERATIONS Enteral and Parenteral

	Date	Comments
(1)		
(2)		

PHARMACIST NOTES and Other Patient Information

	Date	Comments
(1)	8/14	Smoker 2 ppd for 10 years
(2)	8/14	Positive family history for schizophrenia (mother)
(3)	8/14	Positive family history for alcoholism (father)
(4)	8/14	Outpatient medications include fluphenazine; may be compliance problem

1. A proposed mechanism of action of antipsychotic agents is:

   A. Enhanced dopamine release in the locus ceruleus

   B. Increased dopamine reuptake in presynaptic vesicles

   C. Blockade of norepinephrine receptors in the brain

   D. Desensitization of postsynaptic receptors to the effects of serotonin

   E. Blockade of postsynaptic dopaminergic receptors in the brain

2. Antipsychotic therapy for this patient can be assessed by monitoring the target symptom of:

   A. Delusions

   B. Withdrawal

   C. Social incompetence

   D. Apathy

   E. Poor judgment

3. Within 48 hours of initiating haloperidol, the patient experiences uncontrolled and involuntary neck twisting and a fixed upward gaze. The treatment of choice in this patient would be:

   A. Immediate haloperidol dose reduction by one half

   B. Immediate oral administration of bromocriptine 5 mg

   C. Immediate intramuscular (IM) administration of diazepam 5 mg

   D. Immediate IM administration of diphenhydramine 50 mg

   E. Immediate change to an alternative antipsychotic agent such as thioridazine

4. During a patient interview, the physician notices that the patient is having difficulty keeping his legs and feet still. This movement most likely represents:

   A. A dystonic reaction, which may be treated with oral diazepam

   B. Akathisia, which may respond to an oral anticholinergic agent or oral diazepam

   C. Drug-induced parkinsonism, which may respond to oral bromocriptine

   D. A warning sign of reduced seizure threshold; low-dose antiseizure therapy should be initiated

   E. Tardive dyskinesia; the antipsychotic dose should be lowered

5. During a discussion with the patient about compliance, the patient states that he did not like taking oral haloperidol because it made him "stiff." Which of the following can be stated about extrapyramidal symptoms from antipsychotic medications?

   I. Risperidone has a dose-related increase in incidence of extrapyramidal symptoms.

   II. Quetiapine does not have a dose-related increase in extrapyramidal symptoms.

   III. The risk of extrapyramidal symptoms is reduced if the patient's potassium level remains within the normal range.

   A. I only

   B. III only

   C. I and II

   D. II and III

   E. I, II, and III

6. Sexual side effects may affect a patient's compliance with antipsychotic therapy. Which of the following statements is/are correct?

   I. Risperidone and olanzapine decrease prolactin levels.

   II. Prolactin levels are affected by antagonism at the histamine receptor.

   III. Sexual side effects are attributable to an increased prolactin level.

   A. I only

   B. III only

   C. I and II

   D. II and III

   E. I, II, and III

7. Three weeks after discharge on olanzapine 10 mg/day, the patient presents to his outpatient appointment with prominent agitation and delusions. The differential diagnosis includes:

   I. Agitation may be a manifestation of akathisia.

   II. Smoking has decreased serum concentrations of olanzapine.

   III. Early symptoms of neuroleptic malignant syndrome

   A. I only

   B. III only

   C. I and II

   D. II and III

   E. I, II, and III

8. Treatment plans for patients receiving clozapine should include routine monitoring for:

   A. Renal failure
   B. Agranulocytosis
   C. Hair loss
   D. Severe diarrhea
   E. Excessive sodium loss

End of this patient profile; continue with the examination

---

9. When counseling a parent with a 3-year-old on the administration of otic drops to this child, the pharmacist should instruct the parent to pull the ear:

   A. Backward and upward
   B. Backward and downward
   C. 90 degrees outward
   D. Straight forward
   E. None of the above

10. Which of the following agents is the only FDA-approved nonprescription cerumen-softening agent?

   A. Carbamide peroxide
   B. Mineral oil
   C. Hydrogen peroxide
   D. Sweet oil
   E. Glycerin

11. Which of the following would be considered the MOST IMPORTANT counseling point for a patient taking mineral oil?

   A. Remain in an upright position while taking this agent.
   B. Take with food.
   C. It may interfere with the absorption of water-soluble vitamins.
   D. An adult can take up to 3 ounces as a dose.
   E. Do not take if fluid compromised.

12. An older gentleman complains that his hemorrhoids are bothering him again. He has not had problems with them in quite some time. He is concerned because he has noticed that this time around he has had some bleeding into the toilet bowl. What product would you recommend to this elderly gentleman?

   A. Anusol suppositories
   B. Tucks pads
   C. Preparation H ointment
   D. Hydrocortisone ointment
   E. None; he should be referred to a physician

13. A middle-aged woman explains that she has recently developed hemorrhoids and she wants something to stop the itching. Upon checking her profile in the computer, you find out that she is currently taking atenolol 20 mg qd for her hypertension and Lipitor 40 mg qd for her hyperlipidemia. Which of the following would NOT be appropriate for this woman?

   A. Anusol HC-1
   B. Tucks pads (witch hazel, glycerin)
   C. Anusol ointment
   D. Preparation H cream
   E. Hydrocortisone 1% cream

Use the information below to answer questions 14–16.

A 49-year-old woman has recently been diagnosed with rheumatoid arthritis. Bextra was initially prescribed for her condition. She was eventually prescribed Enbrel, and a course of prednisone 5 mg/day was prescribed at the same time.

14. Which of the following apply to the drug valdecoxib in the treatment of rheumatoid arthritis?

   I. This agent works by inhibiting prostaglandin synthesis by decreasing activity of the enzyme cyclooxygenase-2 (COX-2), which results in decreased formation of prostaglandin precursors.
   II. It does not alter the course of rheumatoid arthritis, nor does it prevent joint destruction.
   III. It may cause serious skin reactions.

   A. I only
   B. III only
   C. I and II
   D. II and III
   E. I, II, and III

15. The reason why prednisone is being used in this patient is best described:

    I. As "bridge" therapy to allow the Enbrel to fully take effect
    II. To alter the course of the disease
    III. To minimize the side effects of NSAIDs

    A. I only
    B. III only
    C. I and II
    D. II and III
    E. I, II, and III

16. All of the following apply to the use of Enbrel in this patient EXCEPT:

    A. This agent is used as one of a number of disease-modifying antirheumatic drugs (DMARDs).
    B. It is believed now that agents like Enbrel should be initiated in the rheumatoid arthritis patient within the first 3 months despite good control with NSAIDs.
    C. Inflammatory markers for the disease (i.e., erythrocyte sedimentation rate [ESR]) are reduced significantly by DMARDs (e.g., Enbrel) but not NSAIDs.
    D. It binds to TNF-α and $-\beta$, inhibiting the inflammatory response mediated by immune cells.
    E. None; all of the above apply to the use of Enbrel in this patient.

17. When recommending an appropriate sun protectant for patients, it is important to recommend a product that protects against both UVA and UVB radiation wavelengths. Which agents or combination of agents below would provide such protection?

    I. Titanium dioxide
    II. Octyl methoxycinnamate and avobenzone
    III. Homosalate and Padimate O

    A. I only
    B. III only
    C. I and II
    D. II and III
    E. I, II, and III

18. Which of the following vitamins or minerals would play a role in reducing the risk of neural tube defect birth abnormalities in an unborn child?

    A. Micronutrients such as copper, manganese, and zinc
    B. Niacin
    C. Iodine
    D. Folic acid
    E. Vitamin B12

19. Which statements about cromolyn sodium are true?

    I. Cromolyn sodium inhibits degranulation of sensitized mast cells.
    II. Cromolyn sodium is used for therapy of status asthmaticus.
    III. Cromolyn sodium is the drug of choice for exercise-induced bronchoconstriction.

    A. I only
    B. III only
    C. I and II
    D. II and III
    E. I, II, and III

20. Which of the following would be used to treat antibiotic-associated *Clostridium difficile* colitis?

    I. Clindamycin
    II. Metronidazole
    III. Vancomycin

    A. I and II
    B. I and III
    C. II and III
    D. II only
    E. I, II, and III

Use the patient profile below to answer questions 21–31.

MEDICATION PROFILE—COMMUNITY

Patient Name: John Smith

Address: 14 Francis St

Age: 20   Height: 5'9"

Sex: M   Race: White   Weight: 196 lb

Allergies: Penicillin

DIAGNOSIS

Primary   (1)   Non-Hodgkin's lymphoma

               (2)

Secondary   (1)

               (2)

MEDICATION RECORD Prescription and OTC

	Date	Ɓ No	Physician	Drug and Strength	Quan	Sig	Refills
(1)	6/1	432576	Golub	Cytoxan 1200 mg IV	1	Administer in clinic	0
(2)	6/1	432577	Golub	Vincristine 2 mg IV	1	IV push × 2 min	0
(3)	6/1	432578	Golub	Procarbazine 50 mg	56	iv caps qd × 14 days	0
(4)	6/1	432579	Golub	Prednisone 20 mg	56	40 mg/m² qd × 14 days	0
(5)	6/1	432580	Golub	Torecan 10 mg	10	q 4 h prn nausea	1
(6)	6/1	432581	Golub	Ativan 1 mg	10	q 4 h prn nausea	1
(7)	6/1	432582	Golub	Compazine Suppositories 25 mg	6	i q 6 h prn	1
(8)	6/1	432583	Golub	Neupogen 300 mcg	14	300 mg SQ q AM	0
(9)	6/1	432584	Ferrin	Peridex 16 oz	1	1/2 fl oz bid	1
(10)	6/1	432585	Ferrin	ACT Fluoride Rinse	1	5 weeks swish and spit qd	1
(11)	6/1	432586	Coleman	Hickman Line Kit	1	ut dict	prn
(12)	6/1	432587	Golub	Kytril 1 mg IV over 5 minutes	1	30 min prior to chemo	

PHARMACIST NOTES and Other Patient Information

	Date	Comments
(1)	6/1	Weight 89 kg; body surface area 2.0 m²
		Treatment plan: C-MOPP q 28 days for 6 courses
		Return to clinic 6/8 for CBC and IV chemotherapy
		Cytoxan 600 mg/m²; Oncovin (vincristine) 1 mg/m²; procarbazine 100 mg/m²
		Prednisone 40 mg/m² qd
		Daily Neupogen injections until absolute neutrophil count (ANC) = 10,000

21. All of the following statements about combination cancer chemotherapy regimens are true EXCEPT:

    A. Combination cancer chemotherapy regimens are now used more commonly than single-agent regimens.

    B. Drugs in combination generally should have the same mechanisms of action.

    C. The drugs act during different cell-cycle phases.

    D. The drugs should be associated with different adverse effects.

    E. Cell-cycle–specific agents may be given with cell-cycle–nonspecific agents.

22. Cyclophosphamide is classified as:

    A. An alkylating agent

    B. An antimetabolite

    C. A natural alkaloid

    D. A hormonal agent

    E. A platinum derivative

23. Which chemotherapy agents are associated with a very low (10%) incidence of nausea and vomiting?

    I. Cyclophosphamide
    II. Procarbazine
    III. Vincristine

    A. I only
    B. III only
    C. I and II
    D. II and III
    E. I, II, and III

24. Torecan is a phenothiazine derivative structurally related to:

    I. Compazine
    II. Procarbazine
    III. Ativan

    A. I only
    B. III only
    C. I and II
    D. II and III
    E. I, II, and III

25. To minimize the risk of neurotoxicity, vincristine should be given in doses only up to:

    A. 100 mg
    B. 1 mg
    C. 2 mg
    D. 200 mg
    E. 200 mg

26. What brand-name product should be dispensed for ondansetron?

    A. Velban
    B. Zofran
    C. Kytril
    D. Emetrol
    E. Anzemet

27. All of the following drugs are adrenocorticosteroids EXCEPT:

    A. Prednisone
    B. Decadron
    C. Triamcinolone
    D. Medrol
    E. Provera

28. Which statements describe chemotherapy-induced nausea and vomiting?

    I. Onset of nausea and vomiting usually occurs within 3 to 4 hours after drug administration.
    II. Severe nausea and vomiting may reduce patient tolerance to chemotherapy.
    III. Nausea and vomiting result from stimulation of the brain's chemoreceptor trigger zone (CTZ).

    A. I only
    B. III only
    C. I and II
    D. II and III
    E. I, II, and III

29. Mr. Smith develops a *Staphylococcus aureus* infection at his Hickman catheter site. Because of his history, he is hospitalized for treatment and evaluation. Based on Mr. Smith's profile, which antibiotics would be reasonable therapy choices?

    I. Vancomycin
    II. Dicloxacillin
    III. Unasyn

    A. I only
    B. III only
    C. I and II
    D. II and III
    E. I, II, and III

30. Compazine was ordered for this patient to act as an:

    A. Antipsychotic
    B. Antiemetic
    C. Antidepressant
    D. Anti-inflammatory agent
    E. Antianxiety agent

31. Filgrastim is used to:

    I. Reduce the risk of anemia and certain cancers of the blood
    II. Maintain cell membrane integrity, reduce cellular aging, and inhibit melanoma cell growth
    III. Reduce the risk of neutropenia, which can be life-threatening

    A. I only
    B. III only
    C. I and II
    D. II and III
    E. I, II, and III

Use the information below to answer questions 32–34.

Hydrophilic ointment USP has the following formula:

Methylparaben	0.25 g
Propylparaben	0.15 g
Sodium lauryl sulfate	10 g
Propylene glycol	120 g
Stearyl alcohol	250 g
White petrolatum	370 g
Purified water to make approximately	1000 g

32. Preservatives in hydrophilic ointment include:

    I. Methylparaben and propylparaben
    II. Propylene glycol
    III. Stearyl alcohol

    A. I only
    B. III only
    C. I and II
    D. II and III
    E. I, II, and III

33. How much stearyl alcohol is needed to make 30 g of hydrophilic ointment?

    A. 0.3 g
    B. 1.2 g
    C. 3.7 g
    D. 7.5 g
    E. 8.3 g

34. Hydrophilic ointment is generally classified as:

    A. A hydrocarbon base
    B. An absorption base
    C. A water-removable base
    D. A water-soluble base
    E. A water-insoluble base

35. Which chemotherapeutic agent is most likely to cause nausea and vomiting?

    A. Flutamide
    B. Carboplatin
    C. Cisplatin
    D. Idarubicin
    E. Chlorambucil

36. What patient counseling information should be provided when a patient is prescribed montelukast?

    A. Montelukast should be taken 1 hour before or 2 hours after a meal.
    B. Headache occurs more frequently than in placebo-treated patients.
    C. Asthma symptoms may improve on the first day of treatment.
    D. Worsened allergic rhinitis symptoms may be noted.
    E. Caution should be observed for increased anticoagulation when using montelukast and warfarin concurrently.

37. Which product is most likely to induce hypokalemia in an otherwise normal hypertensive patient?

    A. Dyazide
    B. Vasotec
    C. Aldactazide
    D. HydroDIURIL
    E. Moduretic

38. All of the following are potential advantages of low-molecular-weight heparin (LMWH) over unfractionated heparin EXCEPT:

    A. Increased plasma half-life
    B. Lower incidence of heparin-induced thrombocytopenia
    C. Less risk of osteoporosis
    D. Uses the same monitoring process as for heparin (aPTT)
    E. More predictable dose response

39. Which dosages are available for Zestril tablets?

    I. 2.5 mg
    II. 5 mg
    III. 40 mg

    A. I only
    B. III only
    C. I and II
    D. II and III
    E. I, II, and III

40. Which agent has little value in treating acute inflammation?

    A. Flurbiprofen
    B. Choline salicylate
    C. Acetaminophen
    D. Ecotrin
    E. Ascriptin

41. A theophylline drug interaction potentially exists with:

    I. Lansoprazole
    II. Ciprofloxacin
    III. Cimetidine

    A. I only
    B. III only
    C. I and II
    D. II and III
    E. I, II, and III

42. According to the Henderson-Hasselbalch equation:

$$pH = pKa + \log \frac{[base]}{[salt]}$$

When pKa is equal to 9 and the ratio of the nonionized species to the ionized species is 10:1, the pH equals:

    A. 8
    B. 9
    C. 10
    D. 11
    E. 12

43. Which substance should be used in a case of overdosage with methotrexate?

    A. Brewer's yeast
    B. Leucovorin
    C. *Para*-aminobenzoic acid
    D. Sulfisoxazole
    E. Trimethoprim

44. 5-Fluorouracil is also known as:

    I. FUDR
    II. 5-FC
    III. 5-FU

    A. I only
    B. III only
    C. I and II
    D. II and III
    E. I, II, and III

Use the patient profile below to answer questions 45–59.

MEDICATION PROFILE—COMMUNITY

Patient Name: __Philip Green__

Address: __2127 Sandra Ct.__

Age: __47__   Height: __5'6"__

Sex: __M__   Race: __White__   Weight: __186 lb__

Allergies: __NKA__

DIAGNOSIS

Primary   (1) __Hypertension__

             (2) __Gouty Arthritis__

             (3) __Obesity__

Secondary   (1) _____

             (2) _____

MEDICATION RECORD Prescription and OTC

	Date	R No	Physician	Drug and Strength	Quan	Sig	Refills
(1)	11/21	15776	Melcher	Hydrochlorothiazide 25 mg	30	1 qd am for BP	5
(2)	11/21			Commit lozenge 2 mg	72	as directed	OTC
(3)	12/4	15998	Melcher	Phentermine 18.75 mg	30	1 qd am 1 hr ā br.	3
(4)	1/7	16578	Melcher	Naprosyn 250 mg	20	3 stat, then 1 tid	2
(5)	1/7	16579	Melcher	Lotensin 10 mg	30	1 qd am	6
(6)	1/12			Tylenol 500 mg	100	1-2 prn HA	OTC
(7)	6/22	18967	Melcher	Colchicine 0.5 mg	60	1 bid	2
(8)	7/30	19366	Melcher	Allopurinol 300 mg	30	1 qd am	6

PHARMACIST NOTES and Other Patient Information

	Date	Comments
(1)	1/6	Patient called and states that he has severe pain and swelling in his right big toe that awakened him last night; referred him to his physician for evaluation.
(2)	1/7	Patient states that his MD told him that his serum uric acid was 11.5 mg/dL.
(3)	1/7	D/C hydrochlorothiazide
(4)	1/12	Patient brought aspirin to counter for purchase; advised to use Tylenol instead.

45. Based on Mr. Green's height and weight, he has a BMI of 30. Which of the following statements apply to his situation?

    I. BMI stands for Basal Metabolic Index.

    II. His BMI value meets the definition of obesity

    III. Gradual weight loss would likely lower his serum uric acid.

    A. I only

    B. III only

    C. I and II

    D. II and III

    E. I, II, and III

46. Phentermine should be used cautiously in this patient because:

    I. He has gout.

    II. His BMI is not high enough.

    III. He has elevated blood pressure.

    A. I only

    B. III only

    C. I and II

    D. II and III

    E. I, II, and III

47. While he is waiting to have his phentermine prescription filled, Mr. Green asks, "Is there any safe and effective OTC medication that I can take to treat my obesity?" You reply, "The FDA has ruled that:

    I. no OTC agent is safe and effective."
    II. pseudoephedrine has taken the place of phenylpropanolamine as a safe and effective agent."
    III. benzocaine is effective."

    A. I only
    B. III only
    C. I and II
    D. II and III
    E. I, II, and III

48. Based on the information noted for 1/6 and 1/7, it appears that Mr. Green is suffering from an acute attack of gout. Which of the following descriptions best describes the usual pattern of the arthritis in gout?

    A. Morning stiffness for at least 30 minutes, usually lasting for 1 hour before maximal improvement
    B. Periods of acute attacks with intense pain that completely resolve
    C. Arthritis most commonly in the metacarpophalangeal and proximal interphalangeal joints of the hands
    D. Gradual building of pain over a few days, then a sudden burst of intense pain that typically occurs in the late afternoon
    E. Acute inflammation of two or more joints in a symmetrical pattern

49. The Commit lozenges were recommended for Mr. Green for what purpose?

    I. To help treat his apparent sore throat
    II. As a treatment for an apparent cough
    III. As an aid to help him stop smoking

    A. I only
    B. III only
    C. I and II
    D. II and III
    E. I, II, and III

50. All of the following statements concerning Mr. Green's acute gouty arthritis attack are correct EXCEPT:

    A. Corticosteroids should never be used to treat these attacks.
    B. A good response to colchicine therapy may help confirm the diagnosis of gouty arthritis, but some other forms of arthritis may respond to this agent.
    C. The first attack of gouty arthritis usually involves only one joint; when this is the first metatarsophalangeal joint of the foot, it is termed "podagra."
    D. The patient will likely have an elevated serum uric acid level.
    E. Attacks most typically occur during the middle of the night.

51. Why did the pharmacist advise Mr. Green against taking the occasional aspirin for his headache?

    I. Because in low doses, aspirin can cause retention of uric acid in the body
    II. Because, mg per mg, acetaminophen is much more effective than aspirin for pain from episodic tension-type headache
    III. Because of his increased risk for Reye's syndrome

    A. I only
    B. III only
    C. I and II
    D. II and III
    E. I, II, and III

52. All of the following statements concerning gout or uric acid excretion will apply to Mr. Green EXCEPT:

    A. As a man, Mr. Green is much more likely to develop gout compared to a woman.
    B. Most of Mr. Green's body uric acid is excreted through the gastrointestinal tract.
    C. Foods high in purine content may increase his serum uric acid level.
    D. If he were to take colchicine, it would have no effect on his serum uric acid level.
    E. Naproxen is a good choice over colchicine to treat his acute attack of gout; a justification for this is because diarrhea secondary to colchicine therapy is very common.

53. Mr. Green obtains refills on his Naprosyn for two additional episodes of gouty arthritis. Which of the following would be appropriate considerations in this patient?

    I. With his three attacks, Mr. Green is a candidate for uric acid-lowering therapy.

    II. Small daily doses of oral colchicine would likely benefit this patient by helping to prevent additional attacks of acute gouty arthritis, especially if uric acid therapy is begun.

    III. It would be useful to consider switching him to another antihypertensive, as the current agent may be contributing to his hyperuricemia.

    A. I only
    B. III only
    C. I and II
    D. II and III
    E. I, II, and III

54. Which of the following apply to the allopurinol prescription for Mr. Green?

    I. This drug is known as a xanthine oxidase inhibitor.

    II. He can take this just once daily because of the long half-life of the metabolite.

    III. He must drink plenty of fluids to prevent uric acid crystallization in the urine after starting this drug.

    A. I only
    B. III only
    C. I and II
    D. II and III
    E. I, II, and III

55. Cheryl Green, Philip's wife, comes up to the pharmacy counter and asks you to recommend a vaginal product for her yeast infection. Which of the following would apply to Mrs. Green?

    I. In order to use the OTC agents, she must have had at least one previous episode of vaginal candidiasis that was medically diagnosed.

    II. The OTC vaginal candidiasis products come in 1-, 3-, and 7-day treatment regimens.

    III. The characteristic symptoms of this condition are a vaginal discharge that is described as "cottage cheese-like" with no offensive odor, dysuria, or vulvar or vaginal redness.

    A. I only
    B. III only
    C. I and II
    D. II and III
    E. I, II, and III

56. One of Mr. Green's children, Megan (age 14), developed diarrhea. Which of the following agents are now considered by the FDA to be safe and effective OTC antidiarrheal agents?

    I. Attapulgite
    II. Kaolin
    III. Bismuth subsalicylate

    A. I only
    B. III only
    C. I and II
    D. II and III
    E. I, II, and III

57. You decide to recommend Kaopectate for the treatment of Megan's diarrhea. Which of the following applies to this agent?

    I. This product contains the same ingredient as Pepto-Bismol.

    II. This product should not be given to a teenager who has chickenpox.

    III. Harmless black-stained stools may occur with the administration of this product.

    A. I only
    B. III only
    C. I and II
    D. II and III
    E. I, II, and III

58. A further inquiry into the possible reason for Megan's diarrhea reveals that she seems to get it most often after eating ice cream or other dairy products. You decide against recommending Kaopectate in favor of another product called Dairy Ease. Which of the following can be stated about her condition and your product recommendation?

    I. She probably has lactose intolerance.
    II. Dairy Ease contains lactase, which would be the appropriate agent for treating her.
    III. The diarrhea is caused by the calcium in the dairy products.

    A. I only
    B. III only
    C. I and II
    D. II and III
    E. I, II, and III

59. Ryan (age 13) and Greg (age 15), Mr. Green's other children, are planning to go to the beach with some friends. Mr. Green's family has fair skin, and Mr. Green wants to make sure that his teen sons are protected from the sun. Which of the following would apply to the use of sunscreens for these two teens?

    I. A product with an SPF of 30 or 30+ would provide maximal protection against sunburn.
    II. An adequate amount should be applied, and then it should be reapplied frequently due to loss of sunscreen from sweating or swimming.
    III. The SPF indicates protection against both UVA and UVB radiation.

    A. I only
    B. III only
    C. I and II
    D. II and III
    E. I, II, and III

Use the patient profile below to answer question 60.

MEDICATION PROFILE—COMMUNITY

Patient Name: __Marilyn Fox__
Address: __48 Worthy Rd__
Age: __22__   Height: __5'5"__
Sex: __F__   Race: __White__   Weight: __125 lb__
Allergies: __no known allergies__

DIAGNOSIS
Primary   (1)   Pelvic inflammatory disease
                 (2)   Vaginal candidiasis
Secondary   (1)   Anemia
                 (2)

MEDICATION RECORD Prescription and OTC

	Date	Ṛ No	Physician	Drug and Strength	Quan	Sig	Refills
(1)	9/3	617583	Tacs	Rocephin 250 mg	1	250 mg IM × 1	0
(2)	9/3	617584	Tacs	Tetracycline 500 mg	28	i q 6 h × 14 days	0
(3)	9/3	617585	Tacs	Tylenol with Codeine No. 3	20	i q 4 h prn	1
(4)	9/3		OTC	Feosol	100	i bid	6
(5)	9/7	617843	Greene	Doxycycline 100 mg	30	i tid × 10 days	0
(6)	9/7	617967	Greene	Diflucan 150 mg	1	150 mg po × 1	0
(7)	10/1	618103	Greene	Triphasil-28	28	i qd	12

PHARMACIST NOTES and Other Patient Information

	Date	Comments
(1)	9/7	D/C tetracycline because of gastrointestinal intolerance; change to doxycycline with food (doxycycline is current recommendation of CDC)
(2)		

60. All of the following statements about iron supplementation are correct EXCEPT:

    A. Iron can cause dark discoloration of the stool.

    B. Taking iron with food can decrease absorption.

    C. The usual dose of elemental iron is 200 mg/day in divided doses.

    D. Ferrous gluconate has the highest percentage of elemental iron of all the oral iron salts.

    E. Non-enteric-coated preparations of iron supplements are preferred over enteric-coated products.

61. Mrs. Fox received ONLY one dose, but when dosing fluconazole in patients with renal impairment, which of the following is/are correct?

    I. CrCl > 50 ml/min: no dosage adjustment needed

    II. CrCl 21–50 ml/min: after loading dose, decrease recommended maintenance dose by 75%

    III. CrCl 11–20 ml/min: after loading dose, decrease recommended maintenance dose by 50%

    A. I only

    B. III only

    C. I and III

    D. II and III

    E. I, II, and III

62. All of the following statements about doxy-cycline are correct EXCEPT:

    A. It is active against many gram-positive and gram-negative organisms, My-coplasma, and Chlamydia.
    B. It is mainly excreted in the feces.
    C. Its absorption is increased with concur-rent use of antacids and milk.
    D. It commonly causes gastrointestinal dis-tress.
    E. It may produce phototoxic reactions if the patient is exposed to sunlight.

63. Which products on Mrs. Fox's profile may in-teract adversely with Feosol?

    I. Rocephin
    II. Codeine
    III. Tetracycline

    A. I only
    B. III only
    C. I and II
    D. II and III
    E. I, II, and III

64. Which of the following would most accu-rately describe the antibacterial activity of tetracycline antibiotics?

    I. They are mainly bacteriostatic at normal serum concentrations.
    II. They interfere with protein synthesis by binding to the 30S ribosomal subunit.
    III. They can cause alterations in the bacter-ial cytoplasmic membrane.

    A. I only
    B. III only
    C. I and II
    D. II and III
    E. I, II, and III

65. Which drug is a substituted imidazole for treating many systemic fungal infections and is an effective agent taken orally?

    A. Butoconazole
    B. Clotrimazole
    C. Ketoconazole
    D. Miconazole
    E. Nystatin

66. Chlamydial organisms have been shown to cause pelvic inflammatory disease in some women. Which of the following antimicro-bial agents provide(s) effective therapy for chlamydial infections?

    I. Azithromycin
    II. Doxycycline
    III. Bactrim

    A. I only
    B. III only
    C. I and II
    D. II and III
    E. I, II, and III

67. Which of the following drugs from Mrs. Fox's profile is most likely responsible for her yeast infection?

    A. Tetracycline
    B. Feosol
    C. Triphasil-28
    D. Tylenol with Codeine
    E. None of the above is likely responsible.

68. Based on Mrs. Fox's profile, she has had only one occurrence of vulvovaginal candidiasis.

    Which of the following apply to recurrent vulvovaginal candidiasis?

    I. It would occur if she experienced at least four of these infections in a 12-month pe-riod.
    II. If she had this, she should not try to self-treat with any of the nonprescription products.
    III. This may be an early sign of HIV infec-tion.

    A. I only
    B. III only
    C. I and II
    D. II and III
    E. I, II, and III

69. Mrs. Fox's anemia is apparently due to an iron deficiency. Which of the following would apply to this type of an anemia before treatment with iron supplementation?

    I. One would likely note a microcytic hypochromic blood smear.

    II. The serum hemoglobin (Hgb) and the mean cell volume (MCV) would be low.

    III. The serum total iron-binding capacity (TIBC) would usually be high.

    A. I only
    B. III only
    C. I and II
    D. II and III
    E. I, II, and III

70. Mrs. Fox's initial diagnosis is pelvic inflammatory disease. Which of the following statements would apply to this condition?

    I. This is usually caused by the organisms *Neisseria gonorrhoeae* and *Chlamydia trachomatis.*

    II. The drug regimen of choice for empiric treatment of this condition is ceftriaxone and doxycycline.

    III. The initial administration of Rocephin IM is a rational one.

    A. I only
    B. III only
    C. I and II
    D. II and III
    E. I, II, and III

71. The selection of Diflucan to treat Mrs. Fox's vulvovaginal candidiasis is appropriate because:

    I. It is "less messy" than vaginal creams.

    II. It is considered one of the most effective agents for this condition.

    III. It promotes patient compliance.

    A. I only
    B. III only
    C. I and II
    D. II and III
    E. I, II, and III

Use the patient profile below to answer questions 72–83.

MEDICATION PROFILE—COMMUNITY

Patient Name: _Phyllis Boch_

Address: _68 Ferris Dr_

Age: _34_   Height: _5'4"_

Sex: _F_   Race: _White_   Weight: _110 lb_

Allergies: _Amitriptyline, phenobarbital_

DIAGNOSIS

Primary   (1) _Epilepsy_

           (2) _Mild hypertension_

Secondary (1) _Gastroesophageal reflux disease_

           (2) _____

MEDICATION RECORD Prescription and OTC

	Date	℞ No	Physician	Drug and Strength	Quan	Sig	Refills
(1)	1/5	11238	Dunbar	Dilantin 100 mg	100	iii caps q AM	6
(2)	1/5	11239	Dunbar	Depakote 250 mg	200	ii tabs qid	6
(3)	1/5	11240	Dunbar	Tegretol 200 mg	100	i tab tid	6
(4)	1/30	11473	Huang	Folic acid 1 mg	100	i qd	2
(5)			OTC	Multivitamins	100	i qd	
(6)			OTC	Advil 200 mg	30	ii prn headache	
(7)	2/14	12372	Huang	Atacand HCT 16/12.5	90	i qd	3
(8)	2/14	12373	Huang	Ranitidine 150 mg	60	i qd	6

PHARMACIST NOTES and Other Patient Information

	Date	Comments
(1)	1/10	Dilantin level 16 mcg/ml
(2)	2/4	Nystagmus observed at AM visit

72. Which drugs should be avoided by this patient?

   I. Phenytoin

   II. Primidone

   III. Carbamazepine

   A. I only

   B. III only

   C. I and II

   D. II and III

   E. I, II, and III

73. Ms. Boch has had difficulty swallowing various tablets and capsules. Which medications should she avoid crushing before administration?

   I. Carbamazepine

   II. Folic acid

   III. Depakote

   A. I only

   B. III only

   C. I and II

   D. II and III

   E. I, II, and III

74. Which of the following are common side effects of hormone replacement therapy?

    I. Irregular uterine bleeding
    II. Weight gain
    III. Breast tenderness

    A. I only
    B. III only
    C. I and II
    D. II and III
    E. I, II, and III

75. Therapeutic serum levels of phenytoin are generally considered to be in the range of:

    A. 2–10 µg/ml
    B. 10–20 µg/ml
    C. 15–35 µg/ml
    D. 20–40 µg/ml
    E. 45–65 µg/ml

76. Which drugs decrease hydantoin activity?

    I. Depakote
    II. Folic acid
    III. Tegretol

    A. I only
    B. III only
    C. I and II
    D. II and III
    E. I, II, and III

77. Good oral hygiene is especially important for reducing adverse reactions related to:

    I. Dilantin
    II. Depakote
    III. Tegretol

    A. I only
    B. III only
    C. I and II
    D. II and III
    E. I, II, and III

78. The serum level of Tegretol is unaffected by:

    A. E.E.S.
    B. E-Mycin 333
    C. Amoxil
    D. Isoniazid
    E. Tao

79. Which drug is most likely responsible for Ms. Boch's nystagmus?

    A. Dilantin
    B. Depakote
    C. Tegretol
    D. Folic acid
    E. Advil

80. Dilantin is available as:

    I. A capsule
    II. A tablet
    III. An ampule

    A. I only
    B. III only
    C. I and II
    D. II and III
    E. I, II, and III

81. In addition to hydrochlorothiazide 12.5 mg, Vaseretic 5-12.5 contains:

    A. Ramipril 5 mg
    B. Amlodipine 5mg
    C. Enalapril 5 mg
    D. Quinapril 5 mg
    E. Captopril 12.5 mg

82. The main ingredient in Advil is also the main ingredient in which prescription product?

    A. Motrin
    B. Percodan
    C. Nuprin
    D. Naprosyn
    E. Medipren

83. True comparisons of Advil to Tylenol include:

    I. Tylenol has less anti-inflammatory activity than Advil.
    II. Tylenol is contraindicated in children because they are susceptible to Reye's syndrome.
    III. Tylenol irritates the gastrointestinal tract more than Advil.

    A. I only
    B. III only
    C. I and II
    D. II and III
    E. I, II, and III

End of this patient profile; continue with the examination

84. The brand name for fosphenytoin is:

    A. Dilantin
    B. Cerebyx
    C. Valium
    D. Lamictal
    E. Topamax

85. What type of drug interaction is taking place when reduced blood levels of tetracycline result from taking the drug concurrently with a calcium-containing antacid?

    A. Synergism
    B. Complexation
    C. Chemical antagonism
    D. Electrostatic interaction
    E. Enzyme inhibition

86. Which of the following adverse drug reactions has been reported with the use of quinupristin/dalfopristin?

    A. Photosensitivity
    B. Infusion site pain, erythema or itching
    C. Neutropenia
    D. Cardiomyopathy
    E. Renal failure

87. Naloxone is used in combination with Talwin Nx to:

    I. Decrease the first-pass effects of pentazocine when administered orally
    II. Produce additive analgesic effects with pentazocine when administered orally
    III. Provide narcotic antagonist activity when injected IV

    A. I only
    B. III only
    C. I and II
    D. II and III
    E. I, II, and III

88. If co-trimoxazole oral suspension contains 40 mg trimethoprim and 200 mg sulfamethoxazole per 5 ml, how many milliliters of suspension are required to provide a dose equivalent to one Bactrim DS tablet?

    A. 5 ml
    B. 10 ml
    C. 15 ml
    D. 20 ml
    E. 25 ml

89. All of the following medications are classified as sustained-release theophylline products EXCEPT:

    A. Slo-Phyllin Gyrocaps
    B. Sustaire
    C. Aerolate JR
    D. Accurbron
    E. Theovent

90. Based on a patient's malnutrition and symptoms such as fatigue, weight loss, and paresthesias, the physician suspects pernicious anemia. Which test is the most likely to diagnose this condition?

    A. Schilling test
    B. Hematocrit
    C. Hemoglobin
    D. Serum folate
    E. Schlichter test

91. Which form(s) is/are available for potassium chloride?

    I. Oral solution
    II. Powder in a packet
    III. Liquid

    A. I only
    B. III only
    C. I and II
    D. II and III
    E. I, II, and III

92. What is the side effect most commonly associated with doxazosin?

    A. Hyperkalemia
    B. Postural hypotension
    C. Cough
    D. Taste disturbances
    E. Angioedema

93. All of the following are true of Prilosec OTC EXCEPT:

    A. Available as a 20-mg dose
    B. Available as a purple capsule
    C. Indicated for treatment of frequent heartburn
    D. Patient should not take longer than 14 days without MD direction
    E. Patient should not repeat a 14-day course more often than every 4 months unless directed by MD

94. How long should a patient remain symptom-free on antipsychotic therapy before drug withdrawal is considered?

    A. 4 weeks
    B. 6 weeks
    C. 3 months
    D. 6 months
    E. 12 months

95. Potassium supplementation is contraindicated in patients using:

    A. Chlorthalidone
    B. Hydrochlorothiazide (HCTZ)
    C. Furosemide
    D. Triamterene
    E. Ethacrynic acid

96. To determine the absolute bioavailability of a new controlled-release dosage form of quinidine gluconate, the extent of quinidine bioavailability after the new dosage form should be compared with:

    I. The area under the curve (AUC) after an IV bolus dose of quinidine gluconate
    II. The AUC after a reference standard controlled-release form of quinidine gluconate
    III. The AUC after an oral solution of quinidine gluconate

    A. I only
    B. III only
    C. I and II
    D. II and III
    E. I, II, and III

97. Which is contraindicated in a patient with a history of anaphylaxis related to Thiosulfil Forte administration?

    A. Carbamazepine
    B. Depakote
    C. Dilantin
    D. Acetazolamide
    E. Ethosuximide

Use the patient profile below to answer questions 98–108.

PATIENT RECORD—INSTITUTION/NURSING HOME

Patient Name: __Grace Wiley__
Address: ___57689 South 24th St___
Age: __35___
Sex: ___F___   Race: ___White___   Height: __5'9"___
                                                  Weight: _126 lb__
Allergies: __NKA__

DIAGNOSIS
Primary   (1)   __Bleeding duodenal ulcer__
             (2)   __Hypotension__
Secondary   (1)   _____
             (2)   _____

LAB/DIAGNOSTIC TESTS

	Date	Test		Date	Test
(1)	6/22	Hgb 9 g/dl	(6)	6/22	CO_2 24 mEq/L
(2)	6/22	HCT 30%	(7)	6/22	BUN 25 mg/dl
(3)	6/22	Na 126 mEq/L	(8)	6/22	Creatinine 0.8 mg/dl
(4)	6/22	K 3.4 mEq/L	(9)	6/22	Guaiac-positive
(5)	6/22	Cl 90 mEq/L			

MEDICATION ORDERS Including Parenteral Solutions

	Date	Comments	Route	Sig
(1)	6/22	D5/0.45% NaCl 1000 ml	IV	125 ml/h
(2)	6/22	Al/Mg(OH)$_2$ 30 ml	per NG tube	q 2 h
(3)	6/22	Zantac 50 mg	IV	q 6 h
(4)	6/23	Esomeprazole 40 mg	per NG tube	qd X 10 days
(5)	6/23	Clarithromycin Suspension	per NG tube	500 mg bid X 10 days
(6)	6/23	Amoxicillin Suspension	per NG tube	1 g bid X 10 days
(7)	6/23	D/C antacids, Zantac		

ADDITIONAL ORDERS

	Date	Comments
(1)	6/22	Endoscopy stat
(2)	6/22	Insert NG tube
(3)	6/22	Check *Helicobacter pylori* status (CLO test)

DIETARY CONSIDERATIONS Enteral and Parenteral

	Date	Comments
(1)		
(2)		

PHARMACIST NOTES and Other Patient Information

	Date	Comments
(1)	6/22	Patient has 10 pack-years' history of smoking
(2)	6/22	Patient has recently completed an R_x of ibuprofen for sports injury
(3)	6/22	Open Nexium capsule, administer esomeprazole beads in 50 cc water via NG tube
(4)	6/23	Patient *H. pylori* positive

98. What is the primary reason for selecting an antacid containing both an aluminum salt and a magnesium salt as opposed to a single-ingredient antacid?

    A. Lower cost
    B. A balance of untoward effects such as constipation and diarrhea
    C. Minimal potential for concomitant drug interactions
    D. Better palpability
    E. Decreased frequency of administration

99. Which risk factor is most likely to predispose this patient to the complications of peptic ulcer disease?

    A. Smoking
    B. Race
    C. Age
    D. Sex
    E. *Helicobacter pylori* status

100. Which of the following is/are true regarding *Helicobacter pylori*?

    I. It is present in the majority of patients with duodenal ulcer.
    II. *H. pylori* eradication can cure peptic ulcer disease and reduce ulcer recurrence.
    III. An active duodenal ulcer is best managed with a combination of antisecretory therapy plus appropriate antibiotic(s).

    A. I only
    B. III only
    C. I and II
    D. II and III
    E. I, II, and III

101. In the admission interview, the pharmacist records that the patient has recently completed a regimen of ibuprofen. This information is significant in the patient's history because:

    I. Ibuprofen may cause ulcers even in *H. pylori*-negative individuals.
    II. Ibuprofen may injure the gastric mucosa directly.
    III. Ibuprofen inhibits synthesis of prostaglandins, thereby compromising the mucosal protective effect of these substances.

    A. I only
    B. III only
    C. I and II
    D. II and III
    E. I, II, and III

102. Adding clarithromycin and amoxicillin to omeprazole in this patient will:

    A. Decrease time to symptom relief
    B. Decrease time required to heal the ulcer
    C. Stop bleeding in patients with a bleeding ulcer
    D. Prevent ulcer recurrence
    E. Prevent NSAID-induced ulcers

103. The elimination half-life for ranitidine is approximately 2 hours. What percentage of this drug would be eliminated from the body 4 hours after an IV bolus dose?

    A. 12.5%
    B. 25%
    C. 50%
    D. 75%
    E. 87.5%

104. The binding affinity of cimetidine to the cytochrome P-450 mixed-function oxidase system of the liver may:

   A. Enhance the therapeutic efficacy of cimetidine
   B. Interfere with the metabolism of phenytoin, phenobarbital, diazepam, propranolol, and many other drugs
   C. Decrease the healing rate of duodenal ulcers but not gastric ulcers
   D. Increase the relapse rate of both duodenal and gastric ulcers
   E. Allow for a decreased frequency of cimetidine dosing

105. All of the following reduce acid secretion by inhibiting the proton pump of the parietal cell EXCEPT:

   A. Prevacid
   B. Prilosec
   C. Protonix
   D. Nexium
   E. Pepcid

106. After leaving the hospital, the patient is given prescriptions for Nexium, amoxicillin, and Biaxin to complete the *H. pylori* eradication regimen. The pharmacist dispensed the remaining Biaxin Suspension to avoid waste and minimize the drug costs. You should counsel the patient regarding all of the following EXCEPT:

   A. Continue Nexium 40 mg for a total of 10 days.
   B. Clarithromycin can be given with food to minimize gastrointestinal side effects.
   C. Taste disturbances are common with Biaxin.
   D. Complete a full 10 days of antibiotic/antisecretory therapy for optimal eradication results.
   E. Refrigerate Biaxin, and shake well before use.

107. All of the following are true regarding colloidal bismuth preparations for treatment of ulcer disease EXCEPT:

   A. Bismuth is absorbed after oral administration but is quickly eliminated from the body.
   B. Bismuth products turn the stool black.
   C. The only commercial bismuth product available in the United States useful for ulcer disease is bismuth subsalicylate.
   D. In combination with metronidazole, tetracycline, and antisecretory therapy, they effectively eradicate *H. pylori*.
   E. Pepto-Bismol may cause salicylism when administered in high doses.

108. Which statement(s) concerning the drug misoprostol is/are true?

   I. Misoprostol is effective for protecting patients from NSAID-induced gastric ulcer.
   II. Misoprostol frequently produces dose-related diarrhea.
   III. Misoprostol is contraindicated in women who are pregnant.

   A. I only
   B. III only
   C. I and II
   D. II and III
   E. I, II, and III

Use the information below to answer questions 109–111.

Hydrocortisone acetate	10 mg
Bismuth subgallate	1.75%
Bismuth resorcinol compound	1.2%
Benzoyl benzoate	1.2%
Peruvian balsam	1.8%
Zinc oxide	11%
Suppository base qs ad	2 g

109. The most appropriate suppository base in this preparation is:

   A. Glycerin
   B. Glycerinated gelatin
   C. Polyethylene glycol
   D. Theobroma oil
   E. Surfactant base

110. Bismuth subgallate in this suppository is used as:

    A. An anti-inflammatory agent
    B. A local anesthetic
    C. An astringent
    D. An antiseptic
    E. An emollient

111. How many milligrams of Peruvian balsam are needed to prepare 12 suppositories?

    A. 180
    B. 216
    C. 288
    D. 420
    E. 432

112. The following medication is prescribed:

    Pediazole Suspension 400 ml
    Sig: 2 tsp q 6 h 3 10 d

    Which auxiliary label(s) should be affixed to the prescription bottle?

    I. Take with a full glass of water.
    II. Shake well.
    III. Take with food or milk.

    A. I only
    B. III only
    C. I and II
    D. II and III
    E. I, II, and III

113. Which medication(s) should be labeled "Avoid Alcohol Consumption"?

    I. Dideoxyinosine (DDI)
    II. Metronidazole
    III. Itraconazole

    A. I only
    B. III only
    C. I and II
    D. II and III
    E. I, II, and III

114. Which medication(s) may discolor urine, sweat, and other body fluids and should be discussed as part of patient counseling?

    I. Rifampin
    II. Clofazimine
    III. Atovaquone

    A. I only
    B. III only
    C. I and II
    D. II and III
    E. I, II, and III

115. Which medication(s) is/are frequently in use when nephrotoxicity occurs?

    I. Cisplatin
    II. Foscarnet
    III. Amphotericin B

    A. I only
    B. III only
    C. I and II
    D. II and III
    E. I, II, and III

116. Which condition(s) predispose(s) a patient to toxicity from a highly protein-bound drug?

    I. Hypoalbuminemia
    II. Hepatic disease
    III. Malnutrition

    A. I only
    B. III only
    C. I and II
    D. II and III
    E. I, II, and III

Use the patient profile below to answer questions 117–128.

PATIENT RECORD—INSTITUTION/NURSING HOME

Patient Name: Robert Smith
Address: Sharon View Nursing Home, 98 Colling Rd
Age: 81
Sex: M   Race: White   Height: 5'8"
                                                                   Weight: 175 lb
Allergies: NKA

DIAGNOSIS

Primary   (1)   Pneumonia
              (2)   Asthma
Secondary   (1)   Alzheimer's disease
              (2)   Hypercholesterolemia
              (3)   Hypertension

LAB/DIAGNOSTIC TESTS

	Date	Test		Date	Test
(1)	10/2	Total cholesterol 242	(3)	10/14	Cr 1.4
(2)	10/14	WBC 9.2 10^3 mm³	(4)		

MEDICATION ORDERS Including Parenteral Solutions

	Date	Comments	Route	Sig
(1)	10/1	Advair Diskus	inhalation	ii puffs bid
(2)	10/1	Zafirlukast 20 mg	po	i bid
(3)	10/1	Rosuvastatin 20 mg	po	qd
(4)	10/1	Felodipine 5 mg	po	qd
(5)	10/12	Terbutaline 5 mg	po	i tab tid
(6)	10/15	Cefuroxime 1.5 g	IV	q 8 h
(7)	10/21	Amoxil 500 mg	po	q 8 h
(8)	10/22	Ciprofloxacin 750 mg	po	bid
(9)	10/22	Theo-24 300 mg	po	iii qd AM

ADDITIONAL ORDERS

	Date	Comments
(1)	10/15	Encourage fluids
(2)		Rinse mouth with water after Advair dosing

DIETARY CONSIDERATIONS Enteral and Parenteral

	Date	Comments
(1)	10/1	Low-fat diet
(2)		

PHARMACIST NOTES and Other Patient Information

	Date	Comments
(1)	10/14	Fever to 102.4°F; 10/18 98.6°F
(2)	10/22	D/C Amoxil because rash occurred

117. What is the generic name for Accolate?

    A. Metaproterenol
    B. Albuterol
    C. Ipratropium bromide
    D. Zafirlukast
    E. Cromolyn sodium

118. Which drug is most likely to cause tremor?

    A. Atrovent
    B. Terbutaline
    C. Mandol
    D. Nicotinic acid
    E. Amoxil

119. Which statement(s) concerning cefuroxime is/are true?

    I. It is a first-generation cephalosporin.
    II. It may produce a disulfiram-type reaction if this patient receives alcohol-containing products concurrently.
    III. It is commonly used in patients with community-acquired pneumonia.

    A. I only
    B. III only
    C. I and II
    D. II and III
    E. I, II, and III

120. Which of the following should NOT be used to provide acute relief of bronchospasm?

    A. Albuterol
    B. Pirbuterol
    C. Atrovent
    D. Bitolterol
    E. Proventil

121. All of the following statements concerning amoxicillin are true EXCEPT:

    A. It has an antimicrobial spectrum of activity similar to that of ampicillin.
    B. It is appropriately dosed every 6 hours.
    C. It may cause a generalized erythematous, maculopapular rash in addition to urticarial hypersensitivity.
    D. It produces diarrhea less frequently than does ampicillin.
    E. It is contraindicated in patients with a history of hypersensitivity to cyclacillin.

122. Which agent(s) should Mr. Smith avoid?

    I. Ampicillin
    II. Ciprofloxacin
    III. Erythromycin

    A. I only
    B. III only
    C. I and II
    D. II and III
    E. I, II, and III

123. When using an inhaler a patient should:

    A. Wait 5 minutes between puffs.
    B. Rinse mouth with water between puffs.
    C. Check peak flow readings before and after puffs.
    D. Wait 1 minute between puffs.
    E. Lie down for 10 minutes after dose has been administered.

124. Which agent(s) is/are suitable for this patient's infection?

    I. Cinoxacin
    II. Norfloxacin
    III. Ofloxacin

    A. I only
    B. III only
    C. I and II
    D. II and III
    E. I, II, and III

125. Which statement(s) concerning fever is/are true?

    I. When treating a fever, either acetaminophen or aspirin would be acceptable antipyretic therapy.
    II. Fever is a useful assessment tool; treat only if the fever is dangerously high or the patient experiences chills.
    III. Fever should be treated aggressively; antipyretic therapy should begin on day 1 of antibiotic therapy.

    A. I only
    B. III only
    C. I and II
    D. II and III
    E. I, II, and III

126. Which drug(s) should have serum levels measured and recorded in the patient's medication profile?

    I. Theophylline
    II. Cefuroxime
    III. Terbutaline

    A. I only
    B. III only
    C. I and II
    D. II and III
    E. I, II, and III

127. Crestor is used as an antilipidemic agent to reduce cholesterol. The mechanism of action includes:

    A. Combining with serum cholesterol to form an insoluble complex
    B. Combining with low-density lipoprotein (LDL) in the gastrointestinal tract
    C. Competitively inhibiting HMG-CoA reductase
    D. Combining with bile acids in the intestine
    E. Increasing the metabolism of cholesterol to more polar metabolites

128. The physician would like the patient to use a generic drug product equivalent to Slo-Phyllin. For a generic drug product to be bioequivalent:

    I. Both the generic and the brand-name drug products must be pharmaceutical equivalents.
    II. Both the generic and brand-name drug products must have the same bioavailability.
    III. Both the generic and brand-name drug products must have the same excipients.

    A. I only
    B. III only
    C. I and II
    D. II and III
    E. I, II, and III

End of this patient profile; continue with the examination

---

129. Which of the following is/are thought to shorten the activity of theophylline?

    I. Smoking
    II. Phenobarbital
    III. Cimetidine

    A. I only
    B. III only
    C. I and II
    D. II and III
    E. I, II, and III

130. Procrit is used in chronic renal failure to treat:

    A. Peripheral neuropathy
    B. Anemia
    C. Hyperphosphatemia
    D. Metabolic alkalosis
    E. Hyperuricemia

131. The most common adverse effect of raloxifene is:

    A. Irregular uterine bleeding
    B. Rash and allergic reactions
    C. Hot flashes and leg cramps
    D. Nausea and gastrointestinal upset
    E. Breast tenderness

132. Emulsifying agents can be described as:

    I. Compounds that lower interfacial tension
    II. Molecules that contain a hydrophobic and a hydrophilic functional group
    III. Compounds that have surfactant properties

    A. I only
    B. III only
    C. I and II
    D. II and III
    E. I, II, and III

133. Ketoprofen is structurally considered:

    A. An indoleacetic acid
    B. A propionic acid
    C. An anthranilic acid
    D. A salicylate
    E. A pyrrolopyrrole

134. Which agent(s) interfere(s) with folic acid metabolism?

    I. Trimethoprim
    II. Methotrexate
    III. Pyrimethamine

    A. I only
    B. III only
    C. I and II
    D. II and III
    E. I, II, and III

135. In the preparation shown below, salicylic acid is used for which property?

    Salicylic acid   13.9%
    Zinc chloride   2.7%

    Flexible collodion base qs ad 30 ml

    A. Analgesic
    B. Antipyretic
    C. Astringent
    D. Keratolytic
    E. Rubefacient

136. All of the following agents represent an approved OTC treatment for acne vulgaris EXCEPT:

    A. PROPApH
    B. Liquimat
    C. Rezamid
    D. Carmol-HC
    E. Fostex

137. Which statement(s) about Type I, or insulin-dependent, diabetes mellitus is/are true?

    I. The disease is more common in obese patients over 40 years of age.
    II. The cause of the disease is decreased insulin secretion and peripheral tissue insensitivity to insulin.
    III. Increased serum glucose levels can cause ketoacidosis in these patients.

    A. I only
    B. III only
    C. I and II
    D. II and III
    E. I, II, and III

138. Which type of hormone is represented in the structure below?

    A. Androgen
    B. Estrogen
    C. Glucocorticoid
    D. Mineralocorticoid
    E. Progestin

139. All of the following situations are thought to contribute to the development of Parkinson's disease EXCEPT:

    A. Dopamine deficiency
    B. Norepinephrine deficiency
    C. Gamma-aminobutyric acid (GABA) deficiency
    D. Acetylcholine deficiency
    E. Serotonin deficiency

140. Which combination of antipsychotic agents provides the lowest risk of extrapyramidal side effects?

    A. Tindal and Trilafon
    B. Serentil and Mellaril
    C. Navane and Taractan
    D. Haldol and Moban
    E. Stelazine and Prolixin

PATIENT RECORD—INSTITUTION/NURSING HOME

Patient Name: __Florence Backs__

Address: __2325 Prospect Blvd__

Age: __72__

Sex: __F__   Race: __White__

Allergies: __Penicillin__

Height: __5'5"__

Weight: __158 lb__

DIAGNOSIS

Primary   (1) __Acute pneumonia__

            (2) __Chronic obstructive pulmonary disease__

Secondary   (1) __History of recurrent pneumonia__

            (2) _____

LAB/DIAGNOSTIC TESTS

	Date	Test		Date	Test
(1)	2/28	Chest x-ray (bilateral lower lobe infiltrate)	(4)	2/28	Glucose 124 mg/dl
			(5)	2/28	Albumin 2.5 g/dl
(2)	2/28	WBC 18,000/mm3	(6)	2/28	Arterial blood gases:
		Differential:			pH 7.4
		Segs 80%			PO_2 70 mm Hg
		Bands 10%			PCO_2 45 mm Hg
(3)	2/28	Sodium 140 mEq/L			O_2 saturation 90%
		Potassium 4.0 mEq/L	(7)	2/28	Temperature 102°F (oral)
		Chloride 96 mEq/L	(8)	2/28	Sputum culture and sensitivity
		Bicarbonate 24 mEq/L	(9)	2/28	Theophylline level
		BUN 32 mg/dl			stat = 7.5 mg/ml
		Creatinine 1.4 mg/dl			

MEDICATION ORDERS Including Parenteral Solutions

	Date	Comments	Route	Sig
(1)	2/28	Aminophylline 250 mg	IVPB	stat
(2)	2/28	Aminophylline infusion	IV drip	40 mg/h
(3)	2/28	Acetaminophen 650 mg	po (rectal)	q 4 h prn
(4)	2/28	Ceftazidime 1 g	IVPB	q 8 h
(5)	2/28	Gentamicin 140 mg	IVPB, loading dose	stat
(6)	2/28	Gentamicin 100 mg	IVPB	q 12 h
(7)	2/28	Albuterol 5% nebulizer solution	inhalation	q 4 h prn

ADDITIONAL ORDERS

	Date	Comments
(1)	3/1	Gentamicin peak and trough after third dose
(2)	3/1	Theophylline level (steady state)
(3)	3/2	Cimetidine 300 mg IVPB q 8 h
(4)	3/4	Theophylline level

DIETARY CONSIDERATIONS Enteral and Parenteral

	Date	Comments
(1)		
(2)		

PHARMACIST NOTES and Other Patient Information

	Date	Comments
(1)		
(2)		

141. Based on a volume of distribution of 0.5 L/kg theophylline in this patient, the IV bolus dose of aminophylline would be expected to achieve an initial TOTAL theophylline serum concentration of:

    A. 3.2 µg/ml
    B. 6.9 µg/ml
    C. 10.7 µg/ml
    D. 13.1 µg/ml
    E. 14.4 µg/ml

142. After IV bolus administration, theophylline follows the pharmacokinetics of a two-compartment model. Drugs that exhibit the characteristics of two-compartment pharmacokinetics have:

    I. An initial rapid distribution followed by a slower elimination phase
    II. A rapid distribution and equilibration into highly perfused tissues (central compartment) followed by a slower distribution and equilibration into the peripheral tissues (tissue compartment)
    III. A plasma drug concentration that is the sum of two first-order processes

    A. I only
    B. III only
    C. I and II
    D. II and III
    E. I, II, and III

143. Results of the theophylline level on 3/1 indicate a serum level of 14 µg/ml. Without any change in the theophylline infusion and without any interruption in therapy, the theophylline level on 3/4 was reported as 17.5 µg/ml. Which statement most likely represents the reason for this increase?

    A. The blood drawn for the theophylline level was not timed at steady state.
    B. The blood taken for the theophylline level was drawn from the same arm in which theophylline was infusing.
    C. The presence of ceftazidime in the blood sample caused a falsely elevated theophylline level.
    D. The coadministration of cimetidine competitively blocked the metabolism of theophylline, resulting in a decreased elimination of theophylline.
    E. The patient had a larger than usual volume of distribution for theophylline.

144. After the third dose of gentamicin, levels of the drug were reported as follows:

    Peak, drawn half-hour after ending a half-hour infusion, was 6.2 µg/ml.

    Trough, drawn half-hour before the next dose, was 1.2 µg/ml.

    Gentamicin follows first-order elimination kinetics. Which statement(s) concerning gentamicin pharmacokinetics is/are correct?

    I. The elimination rate constant cannot be calculated.
    II. The elimination half-life can be calculated as 4.65 hours.
    III. If C_{max} is 7.2 µg/ml, the volume of distribution can be calculated as 16.6 L (0.23 L/kg).

    A. I only
    B. III only
    C. I and II
    D. II and III
    E. I, II, and III

145. The culture and sensitivity report for the sputum specimen indicates the following minimum inhibitory concentrations (MICs):

    Ceftazidime < 8 µg/ml
    Mezlocillin < 8 µg/ml
    Gentamicin = 4 µg/ml
    Tobramycin < 0.5 µg/ml
    Ciprofloxacin = 8 µg/ml

    Based on these results, a rational therapeutic decision would be to:

    A. Continue existing regimens without change.
    B. Continue ceftazidime only.
    C. Continue gentamicin; change ceftazidime to mezlocillin.
    D. Change gentamicin to tobramycin; continue ceftazidime.
    E. Change ceftazidime to mezlocillin; discontinue gentamicin.

146. This patient has reported a penicillin allergy. The incidence of cephalosporin–penicillin cross-hypersensitivity is reported to be approximately:

A. 0%

B. 10%

C. 25%

D. 75%

E. 95%

147. The patient has been stabilized on an IV infusion of aminophylline equivalent to 32 mg theophylline per hour. The physician would like to convert the patient to an oral controlled-release theophylline product such as Theo-Dur. Which dosage of Theo-Dur would the pharmacist recommend?

A. 100 mg q 12 h

B. 200 mg q 12 h

C. 300 mg q 12 h

D. 400 mg q 12 h

E. 500 mg q 12 h

148. Which statement(s) about converting this patient from IV to oral sustained-release theophylline therapy is/are true?

I. Considering the theophylline infusion rate of 40 mg/h, conversion to a sustained-release product at 300 mg q 8 h is appropriate.

II. Administration with meals will not significantly decrease the amount of theophylline absorbed.

III. Subsequent theophylline levels should be determined when no doses have been missed in the preceding 48 hours, and the sample should be drawn 3 to 7 hours after the last dose.

A. I only

B. III only

C. I and II

D. II and III

E. I, II, and III

149. The patient would like to receive a generic equivalent of Theo-Dur. In the process of selecting a generic theophylline product, the pharmacist obtains the following information on the generic theophylline product from the pharmaceutical manufacturer:

Eighteen healthy men received either a single oral dose of 300 mg theophylline in controlled-release tablet form or an equal daily dose of 100 mg theophylline elixir given tid. A two-way crossover design was used for this study. In this study, no significant difference was observed in the AUC (0 h–24 h) for serum theophylline concentrations from the tablet compared with the elixir dosage forms. A graph of the plasma drug concentrations versus time was included.

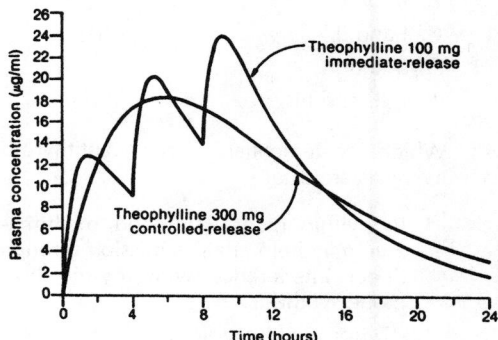

From this study, the pharmacist concludes that:

I. The theophylline tablet demonstrates controlled-release characteristics compared with those of the theophylline elixir.

II. The extent of theophylline bioavailability from both the tablet and the elixir is the same.

III. The theophylline elixir is bioequivalent to the theophylline tablet.

A. I only

B. III only

C. I and II

D. II and III

E. I, II, and III

End of this patient profile; continue with the examination

150. Combivent is a combination of:

    A. Metaproterenol and atropine
    B. Metaproterenol and ipratropium
    C. Albuterol and ipratropium
    D. Albuterol and budesonide
    E. Salmeterol and ipratropium

151. Ingredients with antitussive action that may be found in OTC cough preparations include:

    I. Dextromethorphan
    II. Diphenhydramine
    III. Dihydrocodeinone

    A. I only
    B. III only
    C. I and II
    D. II and III
    E. I, II, and III

152. Which statement(s) about antithyroid agents is/are true?

    I. Propylthiouracil (PTU) and methimazole may help attain remission through direct interference with thyroid hormone synthesis.
    II. PTU or methimazole may be used preoperatively to establish and maintain a euthyroid state until definitive surgery can be performed.
    III. PTU has been associated with serious blood dyscrasias such as agranulocytosis.

    A. I only
    B. III only
    C. I and II
    D. II and III
    E. I, II, and III

153. The belladonna alkaloids are:

    I. Oncovin
    II. Velban
    III. Atropine

    A. I only
    B. III only
    C. I and II
    D. II and III
    E. I, II, and III

154. Metronidazole is effective therapy for all of the following infections EXCEPT:

    A. Amebic dysentery
    B. Giardiasis
    C. Trichomoniasis
    D. *Bacteroides fragilis*
    E. *Escherichia coli*

155. Which statement(s) describe(s) potential problems with drug substances packaged in ampules?

    I. Ampules are made of glass, which can break on opening or during transport.
    II. Drug substances packaged in ampules must be filtered to prevent broken particles of glass from being infused.
    II. Once the ampule is broken open, it must be used; therefore, it cannot be a multiple-dose product.

    A. I only
    B. III only
    C. I and II
    D. II and III
    E. I, II, and III

156. The hypotonic parenteral product is:

    A. Normal saline solution
    B. Half-normal saline solution
    C. 0.9% sodium chloride
    D. Dextrose 40% TPN solution
    E. 3% sodium chloride solution

157. Which infusion method(s) allow(s) reliable administration of a medication with a narrow therapeutic index?

    I. Continuous IV infusion
    II. Intermittent IV infusion
    III. IV bolus with intermittent infusion

    A. I only
    B. III only
    C. I and II
    D. II and III
    E. I, II, and III

Use the patient profile below to answer questions 158–166.

PATIENT RECORD—INSTITUTION/NURSING HOME

Patient Name: _John Stevens_
Address: _Shady Grove Nursing Home_
Age: _81_   Height: _5'9"_
Sex: _M_   Race: _Black_   Weight: _150 lb_
Allergies: _NKA_

DIAGNOSIS

Primary	(1)	Chronic renal failure
	(2)	Dementia
Secondary	(1)	Anemia
	(2)	

LAB/DIAGNOSTIC TESTS

	Date	Test		Date	Test
(1)	5/4	BUN 75 mg/dl	(5)	5/4	Hgb 7.8 g/dl
(2)	5/4	Creatinine 6.0 mg/dl	(6)	5/4	Phosphate 7.6 mg/dl
(3)	5/4	Potassium 7.5 mEq/L	(7)	5/7	Potassium 7.5 mEq/L
(4)	5/4	HCT 24%			

MEDICATION ORDERS Including Parenteral Solutions

	Date	Comments	Route	Sig
(1)	5/4	Mylanta 30 ml	po	prn
(2)	5/4	Kayexalate 30 g	po	qid prn
(3)	5/4	Calcitriol 1 mg	po	i qd
(4)	5/4	Calcium carbonate 1 g	po	ii qid
(5)	5/4	Colace 100 mg	po	bid
(6)	5/7	Haloperidol 1 mg	po	bid
(7)	5/9	Amphojel 30 ml	po	qid pc
(8)	5/9	Ferrous sulfate 300 mg	po	qid pc

ADDITIONAL ORDERS

	Date	Comments
(1)		
(2)		

DIETARY CONSIDERATIONS Enteral and Parenteral

	Date	Comments
(1)	5/4	Protein-restricted diet
(2)		

PHARMACIST NOTES and Other Patient Information

	Date	Comments
(1)	5/9	D/C Mylanta
(2)		

158. Which mechanism describes how Amphojel achieves its therapeutic effect in Mr. Stevens?

    A. Potassium binding
    B. Phosphate binding
    C. Acid neutralizing
    D. Base neutralizing
    E. Ion exchange

159. Kayexalate achieves its therapeutic effect by acting as an exchange resin. Which ion is exchanged with sodium?

    A. Potassium
    B. Phosphorus
    C. Calcium
    D. Nitrogen
    E. Magnesium

160. Which type of anemia is most likely to occur in chronic renal failure?

    A. Normochromic, normocytic
    B. Hypochromic, normocytic
    C. Hypochromic, microcytic
    D. Normochromic, macrocytic
    E. Hypochromic, macrocytic

161. Which medication(s) would need a dosage reduction in renal failure?

    I. Haloperidol
    II. Digoxin
    III. Tobramycin

    A. I only
    B. III only
    C. I and II
    D. II and III
    E. I, II, and III

162. Calcitriol is the same substance as:

    A. Calcium carbonate
    B. Calcium gluconate
    C. 1,25-dihydroxycholecalciferol
    D. Calcium leucovorin
    E. Dihydrotachysterol

163. Which drugs in the patient's therapeutic regimen are likely to cause constipation?

    I. Amphojel
    II. Kayexalate
    III. Calcitriol

    A. I only
    B. III only
    C. I and II
    D. II and III
    E. I, II, and III

164. Life-threatening cardiac arrhythmias due to hyperkalemia should be treated with:

    I. Calcium chloride or calcium gluconate intravenously
    II. Loop diuretics to rapidly eliminate potassium
    III. Sodium polystyrene sulfonate

    A. I only
    B. III only
    C. I and II
    D. II and III
    E. I, II, and III

165. Which adverse effect of haloperidol is most likely to occur in Mr. Stevens?

    A. Neuroleptic malignant syndrome
    B. Extrapyramidal symptoms
    C. Urinary retention
    D. Cardiovascular effects
    E. Decreased seizure threshold

166. When Mr. Stevens complained of gastrointestinal discomfort, the physician prescribed cimetidine. The nurse should be alerted that cimetidine interacts with:

    I. Amphojel
    II. Colace
    III. Ferrous sulfate

    A. I only
    B. III only
    C. I and II
    D. II and III
    E. I, II, and III

Use the patient profile below to answer questions 167–176.

PATIENT RECORD—INSTITUTION/NURSING HOME

Patient Name: ___Mina Peterson___

Address: ___1422 Arlington St___

Age: ___31___

Sex: ___F___   Race: ___White___

Height: ___5'6"___

Weight: ___130 lb___

Allergies: ___Penicillin (rash)___

DIAGNOSIS

Primary	(1)	Acute nonlymphocytic leukemia
	(2)	
Secondary	(1)	Drug-induced congestive heart failure
	(2)	

LAB/DIAGNOSTIC TESTS

	Date	Test		Date	Test
(1)			(5)		
(2)			(6)		
(3)			(7)		
(4)			(8)		

MEDICATION ORDERS Including Parenteral Solutions

	Date	Comments	Route	Sig
(1)	3/5	Cytarabine 200 mg/m^2	IV	qd for 7 days
(2)	3/5	Daunorubicin 45 mg/m^2	IV	qd for 3 days
(3)	3/6	Lorazepam 1 mg	IV	30 min prechemotherapy
(4)	3/6	Dolasetron 1.8 mg/kg	IV	30 min prechemotherapy
(5)	3/6	Dexamethasone 20 mg	IV	30 min prechemotherapy
(6)	3/6	Ortho-Novum 1/50	po	i qd
(7)	3/7	Nystatin Suspension	po	5 ml swish and swallow
(8)	3/7	Cetacaine Spray	to throat	prn
(9)	3/7	Colace 100 mg	po	i tid
(10)	3/7	Gentamicin 100 ml in D5W	IV	i tid

ADDITIONAL ORDERS

	Date	Comments
(1)	3/7	Serum creatinine prior to gentamicin dosing
(2)		

DIETARY CONSIDERATIONS Enteral and Parenteral

	Date	Comments
(1)		
(2)		

PHARMACIST NOTES and Other Patient Information

	Date	Comments
(1)	3/5	Patient has had 3 previous courses of chemotherapy
(2)		

167. Which drug in Ms. Peterson's profile is most likely to cause congestive heart failure?

    A. Cytarabine
    B. Metoclopramide
    C. Dexamethasone
    D. Lorazepam
    E. Daunorubicin

168. The most likely complications seen with Ms. Peterson's chemotherapy include:

    I. Renal failure
    II. Peripheral neuropathy
    III. Alopecia

    A. I only
    B. III only
    C. I and II
    D. II and III
    E. I, II, and III

169. When the second dose of chemotherapy is administered, extravasation occurs. Management of this condition includes all of the following measures EXCEPT:

    A. Leaving the needle in place
    B. Administering potassium chloride
    C. Applying ice
    D. Administering a corticosteroid
    E. Injecting sodium bicarbonate

170. The probable reason for administration of Ortho-Novum 1/50 in this patient is:

    A. Birth control
    B. Estrogen stimulation of white blood cell production
    C. Discontinuation of menstrual bleeding
    D. Progestin stimulation of white blood cell production
    E. Chemotherapy for acute nonlymphocytic leukemia

171. Approximately 10 days after chemotherapy, the cells most commonly affected include:

    I. Granulocytes
    II. Platelets
    III. Erythrocytes

    A. I only
    B. III only
    C. I and II
    D. II and III
    E. I, II, and III

172. In preparing Ms. Peterson's chemotherapy, the pharmacist should take all of the following precautions EXCEPT:

    A. A horizontal laminar flow hood
    B. A surgical gown
    C. Latex gloves
    D. Negative-pressure technique for vials
    E. Syringes with Luer-Lok fittings

173. Nystatin suspension is used as prophylaxis against which organism?

    A. *Histoplasma capsulatum*
    B. *Candida albicans*
    C. *Pneumocystis carinii*
    D. *Pseudomonas aeruginosa*
    E. *Staphylococcus aureus*

174. Ms. Peterson develops a hospital-acquired pneumonia and requires an antibiotic. Which drug should be administered with caution to this patient?

    A. Clindamycin
    B. Tetracycline
    C. Vancomycin
    D. Ceftazidime
    E. Tobramycin

175. Gentamicin is also ordered for Ms. Peterson's infection. The major toxicity(ies) of gentamicin include:

    I. Hepatotoxicity
    II. Neurotoxicity
    III. Nephrotoxicity

    A. I only
    B. III only
    C. I and II
    D. II and III
    E. I, II, and III

176. The FDA-recommended dose of ranitidine to treat gastroesophageal reflux disease is:

    A. 75 mg
    B. 150 mg bid
    C. 300 mg hs
    D. 150 mg qid
    E. 300 mg qid

End of this patient profile; continue with the examination

---

177. Which sign or symptom reflects a vitamin K deficiency?

    A. Dementia
    B. Bleeding
    C. Depression
    D. Dermatitis
    E. Diarrhea

178. Body surface area (BSA) is used in calculating chemotherapy doses because:

    A. BSA is an indicator of tumor cell mass.
    B. BSA correlates with cardiac output.
    C. BSA correlates with gastrointestinal transit time.
    D. The National Cancer Institute requires that BSA be used.
    E. The FDA requires that BSA be used.

179. Aspirin in high doses has been shown to extend the activity of methenamine in the treatment of urinary tract infections. What mechanism is responsible for this drug interaction?

    A. Urinary alkalinization reduces methenamine elimination.
    B. Urinary acidification reduces methenamine elimination.
    C. Urinary alkalinization promotes methenamine elimination.
    D. Urinary acidification promotes methenamine elimination.
    E. Acidification of the gastric contents decreases methenamine absorption.

180. All of the following agents are available as OTC products for the treatment of hemorrhoids EXCEPT:

    A. Steroid-containing products such as full-strength Anusol-HC
    B. Astringent-containing products such as witch hazel and zinc oxide
    C. Local anesthetic-containing products such as Medicone rectal ointment
    D. Vasoconstrictor-containing products such as Pazo or Wyanoids
    E. Aerosol foam products such as Procto-foam

181. Which of the following narcotics has the longest duration of effect?

    A. Methadone
    B. Controlled-release morphine
    C. Levorphanol
    D. Transdermal fentanyl
    E. Dihydromorphone

182. What is the principal ingredient in Burow's solution?

    A. Acetic acid
    B. Aluminum acetate
    C. Boric acid
    D. Sodium hypochlorite
    E. Aluminum hydroxide

183. Which therapeutic agent(s) has been developed from recombinant DNA technology?

    I. Activase
    II. Neupogen
    III. Epogen

    A. I only
    B. III only
    C. I and II
    D. II and III
    E. I, II, and III

184. Effects of the gastrointestinal anticholinergic agent Pro-Banthine include:

    I. Dry mouth, blurred vision, and urinary retention
    II. Increased secretions, diarrhea, and pupillary constriction
    III. Acceleration of gastric emptying time

    A. I only
    B. III only
    C. I and II
    D. II and III
    E. I, II, and III

185. Coumadin should be given with caution to patients in end-stage liver disease because:

    I. Coumadin binding to albumin decreases.
    II. Plasma albumin concentrations decrease.
    III. Prothrombin clotting time increases.

    A. I only
    B. III only
    C. I and II
    D. II and III
    E. I, II, and III

186. A woman has a prescription for 32 mEq KCl po. The pharmacy has 600-mg KCl controlled-release tablets. How many tablets does she need to take each day to provide this dose (mol wt KCl is 74.5)?

    A. Two tablets
    B. Three tablets
    C. Four tablets
    D. Five tablets
    E. Six tablets

Use the information below to answer questions 187–188.

A woman brings the following prescription to the pharmacy after visiting her oncologist:

Carafate 1 g	8 tablets
Sorbitol 70%	40 ml
Vari-Flavors	2 packets
Water qs ad	120 ml
Sig: swish and expectorate	10 ml q 4 h

187. What is the percentage of sucralfate in the final suspension?

    A. 1.0%
    B. 6.7%
    C. 12.4%
    D. 8.0%
    E. 15%

188. How much sucralfate is in 10 ml of this product?

    A. 1.0 g
    B. 500 mg
    C. 66.7 mg
    D. 0.667 g
    E. 6.7 g

189. Passive diffusion of a drug molecule across a cell membrane depends on the:

    I. Lipid solubility of the drug
    II. Extent of ionization of the drug
    III. Concentration difference on either side of the cell membrane

    A. I only
    B. III only
    C. I and II
    D. II and III
    E. I, II, and III

190. Which type of laxative includes the agent psyllium?

    A. Stimulant
    B. Bulk-forming
    C. Emollient
    D. Saline
    E. Lubricant

TEST II ANSWERS AND EXPLANATIONS

1. The answer is E.
The neurochemical basis of schizophrenia appears to be related to dopamine receptor stimulation. Therefore, the therapeutic effect of antipsychotic agents is thought to be related to blockade of postsynaptic dopaminergic receptors in the brain. Other neurotransmitter systems have also been described, but the postsynaptic dopaminergic receptor has received the greatest attention.

2. The answer is A.
Treatment of schizophrenia is primarily symptomatic. Target symptoms of schizophrenia have been categorized as "negative" or "positive" and may be used as a guide in evaluation of therapy. Positive symptoms (e.g., hallucinations, delusions, hostility, hyperactivity) are more likely to respond to antipsychotic therapy. Negative symptoms (e.g., poor judgment, apathy, social incompetence, withdrawal) are less likely to respond to treatment with antipsychotic agents.

3. The answer is D.
An acute dystonic reaction is characterized by involuntary tonic contractions of skeletal muscles of virtually any striated muscle group. The greatest period of risk for such a reaction usually is within the first 24 to 48 hours of initiating an antipsychotic agent; 95% of dystonic reactions have occurred within 96 hours of antipsychotic initiation. Dystonic reactions are more common among patients younger than 40 years of age, and they occur approximately twice as often among men as among women. The reaction is treated initially with an anticholinergic agent such as diphenhydramine, given intramuscularly or intravenously, followed by a short course of oral anticholinergic therapy.

4. The answer is B.
Akathisia is a subjective experience of motor restlessness, and patients usually complain of an inability to sit still. This adverse symptom occurs in approximately 21% to 45% of patients receiving an antipsychotic agent. Onset of akathisia occurs within the first few weeks or months of therapy, and treatment includes lipophilic β-blockers, benzodiazepines, or anticholinergic agents.

5. The answer is C (I, II).
Data from two fixed-dose trials provide evidence of dose-relatedness at doses greater than 4 mg/day for extrapyramidal symptoms (EPS) associated with risperidone (Risperdal) treatment. Quetiapine (Seroquel), at doses from 75 to 750 mg, has evidence for a lack of treatment-emergent EPS and dose-relatedness for EPS. EPS have not been shown to be related to electrolyte levels.

6. The answer is B (III).
Causes of noncompliance are complicated and include poor insight and cognitive deficits. The most manageable cause is undetected adverse effects, such as sexual dysfunction. Sexual dysfunction is secondary to prolactin elevation caused by blockade at the D2 receptor. Presentation may include amenorrhea, galactorrhea, gynecomastia, decreased libido, and erectile or ejaculatory dysfunction. Both risperidone and olanzapine (Zyprexa) elevate prolactin levels. An elevation of prolactin levels was not seen in clinical trials with quetiapine.

7. The answer is C (I, II).
Agitation may indeed be a manifestation of akathisia from his medication. Olanzapine is metabolized by cytochrome P-450 enzymes 1A2 and 2D6, of which 1A2 is induced by smoking. Enzymatic induction may reduce serum concentrations of the target drug, possibly resulting in a loss of efficacy. Clinical signs and symptoms of neuroleptic malignant syndrome are fever, muscle rigidity, altered mental status, and evidence of autonomic instability (irregular pulse or blood pressure, tachycardia, diaphoresis, and cardiac dysrhythmia). Additional signs may include elevated creatinine phosphokinase, myoglobinuria (rhabdomyolysis), and acute renal failure.

8. The answer is B.
Agranulocytosis, defined as a granulocyte count <500/mm³, occurs in association with clozapine use at a cumulative incidence at 1 year of approximately 1.3%. This reaction could prove fatal if it is not detected early and therapy is not interrupted. Patients should have a white blood cell (WBC) count before therapy begins and a clear plan for frequent (weekly), routine WBC assessment throughout therapy.

9. The answer is B.
The objective is to straighten the ear canal so that the drops are easily instilled. In a child, this is accomplished by pulling the ear backward and downward. In an adult patient, the ear canal is straightened by pulling it backward and upward.

10. The answer is A.
Carbamide peroxide is effective in softening, loosening, and helping to remove cerumen from the ear canal. Although the other agents have been used in practice for years, there are no data that support their efficacy above carbamide peroxide in anhydrous glycerin. Sweet oil is another name for olive oil.

11. The answer is A.
Mineral oil (liquid petrolatum) is the only OTC lubricant laxative available. It may rarely be recommended in situations in which a soft stool is warranted, to avoid the patient from straining. In most of these cases, a stool softener would be preferable (i.e., docusate sodium). Lipid pneumonia may result if the patient takes this medication while lying down. It should not be given to bedridden patients. It should be taken on an empty stomach, as taking it with meals will delay gastric emptying. Although the clinical effect is uncertain, mineral oil may decrease the absorption of fat-soluble vitamins A, D, E, and K. The usual dose is 15 to 45 ml (1–3 tablespoonfuls). Patients will not lose fluid with this lubricant laxative as they would with a saline laxative.

12. The answer is E.
Symptoms of hemorrhoids such as burning, discomfort, irritation, inflammation, itching, pain, and swelling can all be treated safely and effectively with various OTC agents. Patients with bleeding, seepage, prolapse, thrombosis, and severe pain should be referred to a physician to rule out a cause other than a hemorrhoid.

13. The answer is D.
All of the above agents would be effective for the treatment of itching from hemorrhoids. Anusol HC-1 contains hydrocortisone, and Anusol ointment contains pramoxine (OTC topical anesthetic). Preparation H Cream contains phenylephrine in addition to shark liver oil, petrolatum, and glycerin. Because drugs absorbed in the anal area go directly into the systemic circulation, this agent might increase the blood pressure in this patient. An appropriate warning label against its use in hypertensive patients is on the product.

14. The answer is E (I, II, and III)
Valdecoxib (Bextra) is a COX-2 inhibitor used for pain and inflammation of rheumatoid arthritis. These agents do not alter the course of the disease, nor do they prevent joint destruction. Warnings concerning postmarketing reports of serious skin reactions and hypersensitivity reaction in patients receiving this drug were issued in November 2002. Patients experiencing a rash while receiving this medication are advised to discontinue the drug immediately.

15. The answer is A (I only).
Low-dose systemic corticosteroids can work well either orally or parenterally for anti-inflammatory and immunosuppressant activity. They do not alter the course of the disease, but they are often used to "bridge" therapy as patients are started on disease-modifying antirheumatic drugs (DMARDs). Corticosteroids will not counteract the side effects of the NSAIDs.

16. The answer is E.
Statements A through D are correct.

17. The answer is C (III only).
Titanium dioxide is a physical sunscreen agent that blocks ultraviolet radiation over both the UVA and UVB spectrum (actually over the entire solar spectrum). Octyl methoxycinnamate blocks UVB radiation and avobenzone blocks UVA radiation, so both spectra are blocked if combined into one product. Homosalate and Padimate O block only UVB radiation.

18. The answer is D.
Increased amounts of folic acid are needed during pregnancy to prevent neural tube defects of the newborn.

19. The answer is A (I).
Cromolyn sodium is used as adjunctive therapy to treat chronic asthma; it should not be used in status asthmaticus. Cromolyn inhibits the degranulation of sensitized mast cells, preventing the release of histamine and other mediators. It is available for inhalation for asthma management in three forms: solution, capsules for use with an inhaler, and aerosol inhaler. Although cromolyn sodium may be used, short acting β-agonists (e.g., albuterol) have shown the greatest efficacy for the management of exercise-induced bronchoconstriction.

20. The answer is C.
Clindamycin is commonly associated with the development of pseudomembranous colitis or *Clostridium difficile* colitis as a side effect. Vancomycin and metronidazole are commonly used to treat antibiotic-associated *C. difficile* colitis when discontinuation of the offending antibiotic does not fully resolve the condition.

21. The answer is B.
Combination cancer chemotherapy regimens are now used more commonly than single-agent therapy and usually involve three or more agents. Combination regimens may have a dramatically higher response rate than single-agent therapy. Drugs given in combination generally should have different mechanisms of action, should act during different cell-cycle phases, should have known activity as single agents, and should be associated with different adverse effects. Cell-cycle–specific drugs may be given in combination with cell-cycle–nonspecific agents.

22. The answer is A.
Cyclophosphamide is an alkylating agent. These agents affix an alkyl group to cellular DNA, causing cross-linking of DNA strands, which triggers cell death. Cell-cycle–nonspecific agents kill nondividing as well as dividing cells.

23. The answer is B (III).
Only vincristine is associated with a very low incidence of nausea and vomiting (<10%). Both cyclophosphamide and procarbazine are associated with relatively high incidences of nausea and vomiting (60–90%), which are caused largely by stimulation of the chemoreceptor trigger zone in the brain.

24. The answer is A (I).
Prochlorperazine (Compazine) is a phenothiazine derivative that is structurally related to thiethylperazine (Torecan). Lorazepam (Ativan) is a benzodiazepine derivative, and procarbazine is structurally unrelated to either.

25. The answer is C.
Administration of vincristine may lead to toxic neurologic effects (e.g., peripheral neuropathy, paresthesias, and ataxia). To minimize the risk of neurotoxicity, vincristine should be given in doses up to 2 mg only.

26. The answer is B.
Ondansetron is the generic name for Zofran. The other products and their brand names are vinblastine (Velban), granisetron (Kytril), phosphorated carbohydrate solution (Emetrol), and dolasetron (Anzemet).

27. The answer is E.
Prednisone (Deltasone), dexamethasone (Decadron), triamcinolone (Aristocort), and methylprednisolone (Medrol) are all adrenocorticosteroids. Medroxyprogesterone (Provera) is a progesterone derivative.

28. The answer is E (I, II, and III).
Nausea and vomiting, common occurrences with many chemotherapeutic drugs, result from stimulation of the brain's chemoreceptor trigger zone. Onset of nausea and vomiting usually occurs within 3 to 4 hours after drug administration. In many cases, symptoms subside in less than 24 hours. A few drugs (e.g., cisplatin) may cause prolonged distress. Severe nausea and vomiting may reduce patient tolerance to treatment regimens. Effective use of antiemetic drug regimens is an important adjunct to successful chemotherapy.

29. The answer is A (I).
Although the three drugs are reliable antistaphylococcal therapy, Mr. Smith's history of penicillin allergy is a contraindication for the use of penicillin derivatives such as dicloxacillin and Unasyn (ampicillin and sulbactam). Vancomycin is not a penicillin derivative and is a valuable alternative for penicillin-sensitive patients. It has excellent activity against *Staphylococcus aureus* (including most methicillin-resistant strains).

30. The answer is B.
Prochlorperazine (Compazine) is a phenothiazine used as an antiemetic agent in cancer patients to control nausea and vomiting, which are common side effects during cancer chemotherapy.

31. The answer is B (III).
Filgrastim (Neupogen) is used to reduce the risks of neutropenic complications in patients with cancer who are receiving myelosuppressive chemotherapy. Potential benefits include a decreased incidence of febrile neutropenia, hospitalization, and antibiotic treatment.

32. The answer is A (I).
Methylparaben and propylparaben are esters of parahydroxybenzoic acid and are common preservatives for both pharmaceutical and cosmetic preparations. Sodium lauryl sulfate is an emulsifier, and the stearyl alcohol acts as an adjuvant emulsifier and adds to the hardness of the ointment. Propylene glycol is hygroscopic and acts as a humectant and cosolvent for water-soluble drugs.

33. The answer is D.

$$\frac{250\ g}{1000\ g} = \frac{X\ g\ stearyl\ alcohol}{30\ g\ total}$$
$$X = 7.5\ g\ stearyl\ alcohol$$

34. The answer is C.
The USP lists four general classes of ointments that are used as vehicles: (1) hydrocarbon bases, represented by white petrolatum and white ointment, (2) absorption bases, represented by hydrophilic petrolatum and cold cream, (3) water-removable bases, represented by hydrophilic ointment, and (4) water-soluble bases, represented by polyethylene glycol ointment. Ophthalmic ointments are listed separately by the USP as ointments for application to the eye.

35. The answer is C.
The incidence of nausea and vomiting with administration of cisplatin is 90%. The other agents listed have a lower incidence of this adverse reaction. Antiemetic regimens should be administered before and during chemotherapy with cisplatin.

36. The answer is C.
Clinical studies have shown that many patients experience an early response to montelukast. Although food may increase absorption of montelukast, the drug may be administered without regard to meal times because it has a wide margin of safety and there are no dose-response effects at doses > 10 mg/day. Headache occurs at about the same frequency as observed in patients receiving placebo, and allergic rhinitis symptoms are not increased. No interaction has been demonstrated with concurrent warfarin administration.

37. The answer is D.
Triamterene–hydrochlorothiazide (HCTZ) [Dyazide], spironolactone–HCTZ (Aldactazide), HCTZ (HydroDIURIL), and amiloride–HCTZ (Moduretic) contain the thiazide diuretic HCTZ, which can cause hypokalemia. However, Dyazide, Aldactazide, and Moduretic also contain a potassium-sparing diuretic, which helps prevent potassium losses. Enalapril (Vasotec) is an angiotensin-converting enzyme inhibitor that inhibits potassium loss from the kidney by inhibiting angiotensin effects.

38. The answer is D.
Low-molecular-weight heparins (LMWHs) (Ardeparin, Dalteparin, enoxaparin) can be given without anticoagulation monitoring because they have a more predictable dose-response relationship. LMWHs have longer half-lives than unfractionated heparin and can be administered subcutaneously with greater bioavailability. LMWHs are also associated with a lower risk of adverse effects typical of heparin such as thrombocytopenia and osteoporosis.

39. The answer is E (I, II, and III).
Zestril and Prinivil brands of lisinopril are available as 2.5-, 5-, 10-, 20-, and 40-mg tablets.

40. The answer is C.
Acetaminophen, a *para*-aminophenol derivative, interferes with prostaglandin synthesis in a manner similar to that of salicylates. However, unlike salicylates, *para*-aminophenols have little value in reducing inflammation. Flurbiprofen is a phenylpropionic acid derivative with analgesic, antipyretic, and anti-inflammatory actions. It may be beneficial in patients with contraindications for salicylates but must be used cautiously in patients with peptic ulcer disease.

41. The answer is E (I, II, and III).
Cimetidine, lansoprazole, and ciprofloxacin all have demonstrated an ability to decrease the clearance of theophylline.

42. The answer is C.
Substitution in the Henderson-Hasselbalch equation gives:
$$pH = 9 + \log 10/1 = 9 + 1 = 10$$
When pH is equal to pKa, the ratio of nonionized to ionized species is 1. When the pK_a is 1 unit above or below the pH, the ratio of nonionized to ionized species is 10:1 or 1:10, respectively. For weak acid drugs, the reverse is true.

43. The answer is B.
Methotrexate (amethopterin, or MTX) is a competitive inhibitor of dihydrofolic acid reductase. Leucovorin (citrovorum factor) is used to neutralize the effects of MTX.

44. The answer is B (III).
5-Fluorouracil is commonly referred to as 5-FU. FUDR is floxuridine; 5-FC is flucytosine.

45. The answer is D (II and III).
BMI stands for Body Mass Index = Weight (lb)/Height (in²) x 703. It is the most commonly used indicator for obesity. Height and weight charts are available to quickly determine this number. A BMI greater than or equal to 30 defines obesity. Gradual weight loss does result in a decrease in serum uric acid.

46. The answer is B (III only).
This agent should be used cautiously in a patient with moderate to severe hypertension. We will assume that Mr. Green has mild hypertension because he is apparently taking only one agent and at a low dose. His BMI of 30 justifies the use of the drug (a BMI of 27 justifies the use of the drug if other risk factors such as hypertension are present). Gout should not be a factor.

47. The answer is A (I only).
The sympathomimetic agent phenylpropanolamine and the topical anesthetic benzocaine were originally ruled as safe and effective OTC weight loss drugs. Because of safety issues (hemorrhagic stroke),

phenylpropanolamine was removed from the OTC drug market. Pseudoephedrine, an oral decongestant that remains on the market for that indication, has not been shown to be an effective weight loss
agent. Because of insufficient evidence of efficacy, the FDA advised manufacturers of benzocaine-
containing products to remove these from the market. The manufacturers have complied, so there are
no safe and effective OTC weight loss agents on the market.

48. The answer is B.
Gouty arthritis attacks occur acutely with complete resolution after a few days. Morning stiffness described above is typical of rheumatoid arthritis. Metacarpophalangeal and proximal interphalangeal
joint involvement is classic for rheumatoid arthritis. Gouty arthritis most commonly affects the first
metatarsophalangeal joint of the big toe. Gouty arthritis attacks typically occur suddenly in the middle
of the night. This scenario matches the pharmacist's note in the profile. Joint inflammation with simul-
taneous involvement of the same joint areas on both sides of the body may be characteristic of rheumatoid arthritis.

49. The answer is B (III only).
Commit lozenges contain nicotine polacrilex (the same ingredient as nicotine gum), which is one of
the newer dosage forms for nicotine replacement. Patients are instructed to use the 2-mg or 4-mg
strength based on the amount of time after awakening when the urge to smoke occurs. Patients who
have this urge within 30 minutes should use the 4-mg product.

50. The answer is A.
Although not generally given as first-line agents, corticosteroids (e.g., oral prednisone) may be used to
treat acute gouty arthritis. NSAIDs and oral colchicine are the usual first-line agents. A positive response
to colchicine may help to confirm the diagnosis of acute gouty arthritis, but other causes of acute arthritis may respond positively to this agent. Selections C, D, and E are all "classic" components of gout.
Mr. Green's presentation per his phone call to the pharmacy matches the descriptions in selections C
and E. Although the serum uric acid is not reported in Mr. Green's profile, it will likely be elevated.

51. The answer is A (I only).
Aspirin in low doses (<2 g/day) inhibits the tubular secretion of uric acid, causing uric acid to be re-
tained. For the treatment of minor pain such as headache, dosages for both aspirin and acetaminophen
are essentially the same. Reye's syndrome, an acute and potentially fatal illness, occurs with rare ex-
ceptions in children younger than 15 years. Fatty liver with encephalopathy develops with this syndrome. The onset most often follows an influenza or chickenpox infection. The risk for this syndrome
increases with salicylate ingestion. Because of Mr. Green's age, he is not at risk for this condition.

52. The answer is B.
By almost a 10:1 margin, gout affects more males than females. Most (about 2/3) of the uric acid excreted by the body is through the kidneys, and this is helpful in using drugs such as probenecid, which
aids in the excretion of uric acid through the kidneys. High-purine foods (i.e., organ meats) should be
avoided, as these may increase serum uric acid levels. Colchicine has no effect on serum uric acid levels. Most clinicians now select NSAIDs over colchicine because of the high incidence of diarrhea from
colchicine.

53. The answer is E (I, II and III).
Initially, acute gouty arthritis attacks resolve completely, usually with no residual effects. The repeated
attacks of gouty arthritis and the fact that his serum uric acid level is elevated would indicate the need
for uric acid-lowering therapy. Prophylactic low doses of colchicine (usually 0.5–1.0 mg/day) may help
to prevent acute attacks of gouty arthritis, especially during the initiation of uric acid-lowering therapy.
Thiazide diuretics (hydrochlorothiazide) may cause hyperuricemia, and switching this patient to a different antihypertensive agent would be appropriate. The use of this agent probably was what initiated
his first attack on 1/6.

54. The answer is C (I and II).
Allopurinol is a xanthine oxidase inhibitor that works to prevent uric acid formation from xanthine. The
long half-life of the main active metabolite (oxypurinol) permits the drug to be dosed just once daily.
Unlike uricosuric agents (probenecid and sulfinpyrazone), which block tubular absorption of uric acid,

resulting in increased amounts of uric acid in the urine, allopurinol actually decreases uric acid formation. Therefore, increased fluid intake is not required as it is with the uricosurics.

55. The answer is E (I, II and III).
To use the OTC agents, a woman must have had this condition once before, must have had it diagnosed by a physician previously, and must experience the same type of symptoms. These agents are available in 1-, 3-, and 7-day regimens. These are all "azole" antifungal agents. The characteristic symptoms are noted above. Other vaginal conditions that are not amenable to OTC treatment will produce symptoms that require medical referral, such as a malodorous discharge, dysuria, and so forth. Patients who experience recurrent vulvovaginal candidiasis infections (four or more over 12 months) should be referred to a physician.

56. The answer is D (II and III).
Kaolin by itself (without pectin), bismuth subsalicylate, and loperamide are now considered safe and effective by the FDA for OTC use for diarrhea. Attapulgite and calcium polycarbophil, which were previously considered safe and effective, were reclassified in April 2003 as Category III agents due to insufficient effectiveness data.

57. The answer is E (I, II, and III).
The trade name product Kaopectate was recently changed to contain bismuth subsalicylate, which is the same active ingredient in Pepto-Bismol. As with other salicylates, these should not be given to children or teenagers with the flu or chickenpox because of the increased risk of Reye's syndrome. A black-stained stool, which is harmless, may occur and should not be confused with melena, which is blood in the stool. Harmless darkening of the tongue can also occur with bismuth subsalicylate use.

58. The answer is C (I and II).
Lactose intolerance is relatively common. Disaccharides, like lactose and sucrose, are normally hydrolyzed by lactase. If lactase is not present, these disaccharides may produce an osmotic diarrhea. Products such as Dairy Ease, which contain lactase, can be administered before eating dairy products to relieve this problem. Also, lactose-free milk products can be used in place of regular milk. Calcium, although probably not in the doses present in various dairy products, will eventually cause constipation, not diarrhea.

59. The answer is C (I and II).
An SPF (Sun Protection Factor) of 30 blocks about 97% of UVB radiation and would certainly provide maximal protection against sunburn. Any benefit from using SPFs above 30 would be negligible. All sun-exposed surfaces should be covered liberally and evenly. An average-sized adult in a swimsuit would require about 1 oz. application. Perspiration, swimming, and toweling off all contribute to the need for reapplication. The SPF is a measure of only UVB protection. UVA radiation, which is relatively constant throughout the day, is not blocked by sunscreen agents that are limited to the UVB spectrum. The sunscreen agent Avobenzone blocks most of the UVA rays.

60. The answer is D.
Ferrous sulfate and fumarate have higher percentages of elemental iron than the gluconate salt. Enteric-coated formulations do not dissolve until they enter the small intestine, which causes a reduction in iron absorption. Items A, B, and C are all correct statements concerning iron supplementation.

61. The answer is A.
For a CrCl > 50 ml/min, no dosage change is necessary. For a CrCl 21–50 ml/min, the recommended maintenance dose should be decreased by 50%. For a CrCl of 11–20, the recommended maintenance dose should be decreased by 75%.

62. The answer is C.
Tetracyclines are broad-spectrum agents effective against gram-negative and gram-positive organisms, spirochetes, Mycoplasma and Chlamydia organisms, rickettsial species, and certain protozoa. Because doxycycline is excreted mainly in the feces, it is the safest tetracycline for treatment of extrarenal infections in patients with renal impairment. Phototoxic reactions (enhanced sunburn) can develop with exposure to sunlight. Doxycycline has the least binding affinity for Ca^{++} ions of any of the tetracyclines,

but the net effect is a slight decrease in absorption, not an increase. Unlike other tetracycline derivatives, food and/or antacids do not significantly inhibit absorption of doxycycline. Gastrointestinal distress is a common adverse effect of all tetracyclines; it may be minimized by concurrent administration with food.

63. The answer is B (III).
Iron preparations form a chelate with tetracycline, inhibiting its absorption; therefore, iron preparations should not be administered with oral tetracyclines. If a patient needs both types of therapy, the iron product should be administered 3 hours before or 2 hours after the tetracycline to minimize the adverse interaction.

64. The answer is E (I, II, and III).
Tetracyclines are mainly bacteriostatic, but at high concentrations they can be bactericidal. They inhibit bacterial protein synthesis by binding to the 30S ribosomal subunit, thus interfering with the transfer of genetic information. They can also inhibit the bacterial cytoplasmic membrane, reducing membrane stability and thus causing bacterial cell lysis.

65. The answer is C.
Ketoconazole is an oral agent effective for treating systemic fungal infections. Butoconazole, clotrimazole, and miconazole are administered topically or vaginally for local infection. Nystatin is a polyene antifungal antibiotic, not a substituted imidazole derivative. It is available for topical and vaginal administration to treat local infections. Nystatin oral tablets are not absorbed and are therefore therapeutic only for infections of the gastrointestinal tract, especially oral and esophageal *Candida* infections.

66. The answer is C.
Azithromycin and doxycycline are the drugs of choice for treatment of chlamydial infections. Sulfonamide products (including Bactrim) are neither appropriate nor reliable for treating infections caused by Chlamydial organisms.

67. The answer is A.
Tetracycline and other broad-spectrum antibiotics are a common cause for vulvovaginal candidiasis. Estrogen-containing oral contraceptives (e.g., Triphasil-28) might cause this problem, but it was started after the candida infection. The other agents, ferrous sulfate and Tylenol with Codeine, are not associated with the development of this infection.

68. The answer is E (I, II, and III).
Patients who experience these recurrent vulvovaginal candidiasis infections may be experiencing a mixed infection or a strain of candidal infection other than *C. albicans*. These infections might be resistant to standard therapy. All of the above items are correct.

69. The answer is E (I, II, and III).
Iron deficiency anemia usually produces a microcytic hypochromic type of anemia. The red blood cells are smaller and lighter in color than normal. The hemoglobin level in the blood will be low. Red blood cell indices such as the mean cell volume (MCV) and the mean cell hemoglobin concentration (MCHC) will both be low, reflecting the microcytic and hypochromic nature of the red cells. Total iron-binding capacity will be high.

70. The answer is E (I, II, and III).
Common organisms that can cause pelvic inflammatory disease include *Neisseria gonorrhoeae* and *Chlamydia trachomatis*. Empiric treatment is therefore directed toward eradicating these organisms. Empiric treatment uses a combination regimen of ceftriaxone (Rocephin) given intramuscularly once followed by an oral tetracycline antibiotic (e.g., doxycycline or tetracycline) given for 10 to 14 days.

71. The answer is E (I, II, and III).
Single-dose oral fluconazole has been shown to have clinical efficacy as good as or better than topical antifungal products. Because it can be given as a single oral tablet, it is considered "cleaner" than topical agents, many of which need to be dosed three or more times to reach the efficacy afforded by one oral dose of fluconazole. These factors have both led to improved patient compliance.

72. The answer is D (II, III).
Phenytoin, primidone, and carbamazepine are all agents indicated for treatment of generalized tonic–clonic seizures. Primidone metabolizes to phenobarbital; therefore, patients who are allergic to phenobarbital should not receive primidone. Carbamazepine is contraindicated in patients with hypersensitivity to tricyclic antidepressants, such as amitriptyline.

73. The answer is B (III).
Depakote is an enteric-coated preparation of valproic acid and should not be crushed. All enteric-coated products must remain intact to prevent dissolution in the stomach.

74. The answer is E (I, II, and III).
As many as 54% to 86% of women receiving hormone replacement therapy (estrogen–progestin replacement therapy) will experience irregular uterine bleeding. Other adverse effects include breast tenderness, headache, nausea, and weight gain.

75. The answer is B.
The normal therapeutic range for phenytoin serum levels is 10 to 20 mg/ml. Nystagmus, ataxia, and slurred speech have been reported with serum levels of 20 to 30 mg/ml, with coma reported when the level reaches 40 mg/ml.

76. The answer is D (II, III).
Folic acid enhances phenytoin (hydantoin) clearance, which can result in reduced phenytoin serum levels and loss of efficacy. Carbamazepine (Tegretol) may also enhance phenytoin metabolism and thus reduce plasma phenytoin levels and therapeutic efficacy. Phenytoin has the same effect on carbamazepine.

77. The answer is A (I).
Good oral hygiene, including gum massage, frequent brushing and flossing, and appropriate dental care, may decrease gingival hyperplasia related to phenytoin (Dilantin) use.

78. The answer is C.
Penicillins such as Amoxil have not been shown to affect carbamazepine (Tegretol) levels. Erythromycin (E.E.S. or E-Mycin 333), isoniazid (Laniazid), and troleandomycin (Tao) all have reportedly increased Tegretol levels.

79. The answer is A.
Nystagmus is an early sign of phenytoin (Dilantin) intoxication. Other reactions common with phenytoin use are confusion, slurred speech, drowsiness, and ataxia. All are dose-related adverse effects involving the central nervous system.

80. The answer is E (I, II, and III).
Phenytoin sodium (Dilantin) is available as a capsule, as a tablet, and as an ampule for IV administration.

81. The answer is C.
Vaseretic 5-12.5 contains enalapril 5 mg and hydrochlorothiazide (HCTZ) 12.5 mg.

82. The answer is A.
Advil, Nuprin, and Medipren contain 200 mg ibuprofen and may be sold OTC. Motrin and Rufen contain at least 400 mg ibuprofen and can be sold only with a prescription. Naproxen (Naprosyn) is an NSAID. Percodan is the brand name for oxycodone, a narcotic analgesic.

83. The answer is A (I).
Acetaminophen (Tylenol) has analgesic and antipyretic activity but very little anti-inflammatory activity. Aspirin, not acetaminophen, is contraindicated in small children with fever due to a viral infection because they are susceptible to Reye's syndrome.

84. The answer is B.
The brand name for fosphenytoin is Cerebyx. Other brand names are phenytoin (Dilantin), diazepam (Valium), lamotrigine (Lamictal), and topiramate (Topamax).

85. The answer is B.
When tetracycline is administered with a calcium-containing antacid, a complex is formed that reduces the absorption of tetracycline. Synergism is an example of potentiation of one drug's interaction with another; for example, when aminoglycosides are combined with agents such as mezlocillin, their combined effect is greater than the addition of each individual effect. Competitive antagonism results when two agents compete for the same receptor site, such as when atropine sulfate competes with acetylcholine for the cholinergic receptor site.

86. The answer is B.
Reported adverse drug reactions with quinupristin/dalfopristin (Synercid) are generally mild and infusion-related: pain, erythema, or itching at the infusion site, increases in pulse and diastolic blood pressure, headache, nausea or vomiting, and diarrhea. Synercid does not alter hematologic or renal indices, but it may increase liver function tests slightly.

87. The answer is B (III).
Naloxone, which is a pure opioid antagonist, reverses or prevents the effects of opioids but has no opioid-receptor agonist activity. Naloxone is not absorbed after oral administration; however, after IV administration, it blocks the pharmacologic effects of pentazocine (Talwin), producing withdrawal symptoms in opioid-dependent persons.

88. The answer is D.
Bactrim DS contains 160 mg trimethoprim and 800 mg sulfamethoxazole. Twenty milliliters of co-trimoxazole suspension would be required to provide an equivalent dose.

89. The answer is D.
Accurbron is the brand name for a theophylline liquid preparation. Slo-Phyllin Gyrocaps, Sustaire, Aerolate JR, and Theovent are theophylline sustained-release preparations.

90. The answer is A.
The Schilling test is used to diagnose pernicious anemia, or vitamin B12 deficiency. Hematocrit, hemoglobin, and serum folate measurements are not specific for B12 deficiency. The Schlichter test is used in bacterial endocarditis to ensure adequate antibiotic concentration in the blood.

91. The answer is E (I, II, and III).
Potassium chloride is available as an oral solution, as a powder, and as a liquid to be given by IV injection. For ambulatory use, potassium chloride is available as an oral solution, or as a powder in a packet to be mixed with water or juice. The injection form is for rapid IV potassium repletion or as an addition to total parenteral nutrition (TPN).

92. The answer is B.
Postural hypotension is commonly experienced with α1-blockers, including doxazosin, because of the direct action.

93. The answer is B.
Prilosec OTC is available as salmon-colored tablets; prescription Prilosec 20 mg is available as purple capsules.

94. The answer is D.
Maintenance antipsychotic therapy is intended to prevent relapse. Usually it is suggested that the patient remain symptom-free for 6 months before therapy is discontinued. Discontinuing therapy should be tried with the patient's willingness and should be accomplished through dosage tapering. Relapse during dose tapering would be likely to preclude therapy discontinuation.

95. The answer is D.
Hyperkalemia is a major risk with potassium-sparing diuretics, and potassium supplementation is therefore contraindicated. To reduce the risk of hyperkalemia, the patient may use a combination of diuretic products such as Dyazide (triamterene with hydrochlorothiazide [HCTZ]), Aldactazide (spironolactone with HCTZ), or other combinations.

96. The answer is A (I).
Absolute bioavailability is a measurement of the fraction of the dose that is systemically absorbed. To estimate absolute bioavailability, the area under the curve (AUC) after the drug product is given orally is compared with the AUC after an IV bolus dose, because only the IV bolus dose is known to be 100% absorbed. Relative bioavailability compares the AUC of one dosage form with that of another dosage form, usually a drug solution or reference drug product given by the same route of administration.

97. The answer is D.
Acetazolamide (Diamox) is a carbonic anhydrase inhibitor and a nonbacteriostatic sulfonamide derivative. Sulfamethizole (Thiosulfil Forte) is a sulfonamide antibiotic. Therefore, cross-sensitivity may exist between these drugs.

98. The answer is B.
Antacids, which act to neutralize gastric acids, are available primarily as magnesium, aluminum, calcium, or sodium salts. A product that is a combination of magnesium and aluminum salts permits a lower dosage of each compound. In addition, with such a combination, the constipating effect of the aluminum salt counteracts the laxative effect of the magnesium salt, thereby minimizing the consequences of each compound.

99. The answer is E.
A number of risk factors are associated with peptic ulcer disease, but the dominant causative factor is *Helicobacter pylori* infection. Eradication of *H. pylori* infection can cure peptic ulcers in many patients and prevent rebleeding in patients like this one. Alcohol, NSAIDs, corticosteroids, and coffee drinking also are included as risk factors, as is cigarette smoking. These factors contribute to risk to a lesser degree than *H. pylori*. In addition, ulcer healing is delayed in a patient who smokes, and the risk and rapidity of relapse are both increased after the ulcer has healed. Smoking accelerates the emptying of stomach acid into the duodenum.

100. The answer is E (I, II, and III).
Helicobacter pylori infection is present in the majority of duodenal ulcer patients. The major benefit to eradication of the infection is prevention of recurrent ulcer disease. Ulcers recur in more than 80% of *H. pylori*-positive patients whose duodenal ulcers are healed within 1 year. Eradication prevents recurrence in most patients and may eliminate the need for maintenance antisecretory therapy. Treatment of active duodenal ulcers is best managed with a combination of antisecretory agents to relieve symptoms and heal the ulcer, and appropriate antibiotics to eradicate the infection and prevent recurrence.

101. The answer is E (I, II, and III).
NSAIDs such as ibuprofen are inhibitors of prostaglandin synthesis. Although the inhibition is an important mechanism for anti-inflammatory therapy, it also compromises the protective effects that prostaglandins exert on the gastric mucosa. NSAIDs can also injure the gastric mucosa directly by allowing back-diffusion of hydrogen ions into the mucosa. NSAIDs are independent risk factors for peptic ulcer disease and can cause ulcers in *Helicobacter pylori*-negative patients. In fact, NSAIDs are the principal cause of ulcers in patients who are not infected.

102. The answer is D.
The addition of clarithromycin to this patient's regimen is intended to prevent ulcer recurrence and rebleeding. Symptom resolution and ulcer healing are produced by the antisecretory therapy (omeprazole), and efficacy for these outcomes is not changed by addition of the antibiotic. Neither drug seems to stop bleeding, although it is believed that increasing intragastric pH with antisecretory agents may improve clotting. NSAIDs are independent risk factors for ulcers, and eradication of the infection does not prevent ulcers caused by NSAIDs.

103. The answer is D.
For any first-order process, 50% of the initial amount of drug is eliminated at the end of the first half-life, and 50% of the remaining amount of drug (i.e., 75% of the original amount) is eliminated at the end of the second half-life. The half-life for ranitidine is about 2 hours; therefore, in 2 hours 50% of the drug is eliminated, and in 4 hours 75% of the drug is eliminated.

104. The answer is B.
Cimetidine is known to bind to the cytochrome P-450 mixed-function oxidative pathway of the liver. This binding affinity may interfere with the metabolism of other agents dependent on this route of clearance. These agents include phenytoin, theophylline, phenobarbital, lidocaine, warfarin, imipramine, diazepam, and propranolol.

105. The answer is E.
Prevacid (lansoprazole), Prilosec (omeprazole), Protonix (pantoprazole), and Nexium (esomeprazole) are proton pump inhibitors. Pepcid (famotidine) is an H2-receptor antagonist.

106. The answer is E.
Biaxin Suspension should be stored at room temperature. It should be shaken well before use. Appropriate advice for the patient should include recommendations to take the complete 10 days of antibiotics required for eradication, together with Nexium 40 mg daily. Finally, administration of clarithromycin with food may minimize gastrointestinal complaints.

107. The answer is A.
Bismuth is not well absorbed after administration of bismuth subsalicylate or bismuth subcitrate. Only bismuth subsalicylate (Pepto-Bismol) is available in the United States. Bismuth compounds discolor the stool black; this may alarm patients because black stools may also be a sign of blood (gastrointestinal bleeding). Bismuth compounds have been effectively combined with antibiotics and antisecretory compounds to eradicate *Helicobacter pylori.* Large doses of bismuth subsalicylate may cause salicylism.

108. The answer is E (I, II, and III).
Misoprostol is the only agent approved to protect patients from NSAID-induced gastric ulcers. Misoprostol is a synthetic prostaglandin that appears to suppress gastric acid secretion and may provide a mucosal protective effect. It is used in patients taking NSAID therapy to counter the undesired effect that these compounds exert on prostaglandin activity in the parietal cell of the gastric mucosa. Misoprostol is contraindicated in pregnant women because it may induce spontaneous uterine contractions.

109. The answer is D.
Theobroma oil (cocoa butter) is a mixed triglyceride suppository base that melts at 34°to 35°C. Its emollient and nonirritating characteristics allow its use as a base for hemorrhoidal suppositories. Glycerinated gelatin suppositories are used as vaginal suppositories for the local application of antibacterial agents. Glycerin or soap suppositories contain sodium stearate, which is used for its laxative effect. Polyethylene glycol bases are water-miscible suppository bases used with various drugs for systemic absorption.

110. The answer is C.
Bismuth subgallate and zinc oxide are astringents to close capillaries and prevent bleeding.

111. The answer is E.
The amount of Peruvian balsam in one suppository (2 g) is equal to 0.018×2000 mg; therefore, for 12 suppositories:

$$0.018 \times \frac{2000 \text{ mg}}{\text{suppositories}} \times 12 \text{ suppositories} = 432 \text{ mg}$$

112. The answer is C (I, II).
Pediazole Suspension (erythromycin and sulfisoxazole) requires proper shaking before each dose. As with other sulfonamides, a full glass of water is recommended with each dose to ensure adequate hydration to minimize the risk of crystalluria.

113. The answer is C (I, II).
Patients receiving metronidazole may experience a disulfiram-type reaction if they consume alcohol concurrently with the drug. Tachycardia and flushing may occur if alcohol is consumed during dideoxyinosine (DDI) therapy. The use of DDI and alcohol should be avoided because of the potential for drug-induced pancreatitis. These reactions have not been reported in patients receiving itraconazole.

114. The answer is C (I, II).
Rifampin colors urine, sweat, tears, saliva, and feces orange-red. Clofazimine may discolor urine, sweat, and other body fluids pink to brownish. Clofazimine produces pink to brownish skin pigmentation in 75% to 100% of patients within a few weeks. The skin discoloration has led to severe depression in some patients. Atovaquone produces no body fluid discoloration or skin pigmentation.

115. The answer is E (I, II, and III).
Cisplatin, foscarnet, and amphotericin B can cause nephrotoxicity. Renal function tests should be performed and serum creatinine levels and blood urea nitrogen (BUN) should be monitored when these medications are administered.

116. The answer is E (I, II, and III).
Although the theory is controversial, it is thought that drugs that are highly bound to albumin will have higher concentrations of free drug circulating in the blood if albumin levels are reduced. Hypoalbuminemia, liver (hepatic) disease, malnutrition, and cancer are several of the more common conditions that result in decreased albumin levels, which necessitate alterations in dosage in highly albumin-bound drugs.

117. The answer is D.
The generic name for Accolate is zafirlukast. It is a leukotriene receptor antagonist used for the prophylaxis and treatment of asthma.

118. The answer is B.
Tremor is often the dose-limiting side effect related to terbutaline use. Tremor also has been reported to occur with other sympathomimetic drugs.

119. The answer is B (III).
Cefuroxime (Ceftin, Kefurox, Zinacef) is a second-generation cephalosporin. Alcohol consumption can result in a disulfiram-type reaction in patients receiving cefamandole (or the third-generation agents moxalactam and cefoperazone), but this does not occur with cefuroxime. Cefuroxime often is prescribed as an alternative to ampicillin (as is cefamandole) to treat community-acquired pneumonia and is administered in a dosage of 2.25 to 4.5 g per day, which is divided and given every 8 hours. All cephalosporins should be used cautiously in penicillin-allergic patients.

120. The answer is C.
Atrovent (ipratropium) should not be used for symptom relief or for exacerbations of bronchospasm. The onset of action is within 15 minutes, and the agent is useful mainly for maintenance regimens in patients with COPD and some patients with asthma. The other agents listed have more rapid onsets (within 5 minutes) and are useful to relieve acute bronchospasm.

121. The answer is B.
Amoxicillin has a spectrum of antimicrobial activity similar to that of ampicillin. It has a longer half-life, which allows less frequent dosing (250–500 mg every 8 hours, as opposed to ampicillin, which is given in a dosage of 250 mg–2 g every 4–6 hours). Both drugs may produce an erythematous, maculopapular rash not seen with other penicillins. Amoxicillin has more complete oral absorption than ampicillin—a characteristic that may explain the lower frequency of diarrhea as a side effect. It is contraindicated in patients with a history of hypersensitivity to other penicillins.

122. The answer is A (I).
With this patient's recent history of rash caused by amoxicillin, ampicillin should be avoided because an erythematous, maculopapular rash or an urticarial hypersensitivity is seen with other penicillins.

Ciprofloxacin and erythromycin are both reasonable alternatives in terms of the potential interaction of these agents with theophylline (Slo-Phyllin).

123. The answer is D.
For optimal dose retention, patients should be instructed to wait 1 minute between each puff. Longer waits between puffs are unnecessary and may contribute to nonadherence to the prescribed regimen. Patients using steroid inhalers, especially, should be instructed to rinse well after completing their dosing. If the immediate response to an inhaled β-agonist needs to be documented, patients should wait until all of their puffs have been administered before checking their peak flows. Lying down is unnecessary following administration of inhaled agents.

124. The answer is B (III).
Only ofloxacin (Floxin) is suitable for systemic infections such as pneumonia. Cinoxacin and norfloxacin are indicated only for urinary tract infections.

125. The answer is C (I, II).
Fever is an important monitoring parameter in infectious diseases; however, administration of antipyretics masks fever. Subsidence of a fever (defervescence) usually indicates a favorable response to therapy. Fever should be treated only if the patient has chills or if the fever is dangerously high. If needed, acetaminophen or aspirin is acceptable. Because fever sometimes stems from noninfectious conditions that do not respond to antibiotics (e.g., metabolic disorders, drug reactions, and neoplasms), fever should not be treated with anti-infective agents unless infection has been identified as the cause.

126. The answer is A (I).
Of the medications that this patient is receiving, only theophylline levels are commonly measured. These tests are available through commercial clinical laboratories.

127. The answer is C.
Zocor (simvastatin) is a competitive inhibitor of the enzyme HMG-CoA reductase, the enzyme that catalyzes the early rate-limiting step in cholesterol biosynthesis. HMG-CoA reductase inhibitors increase high-density lipoprotein (HDL) cholesterol and decrease low-density lipoprotein (LDL) cholesterol, very low-density lipoprotein (VLDL) cholesterol, and plasma triglycerides. Other HMG-CoA reductase inhibitors include lovastatin (Mevacor), pravastatin (Pravachol), fluvastatin (Lescol), cerivastatin (Baycol), and atorvastatin (Lipitor).

128. The answer is C (I, II).
Bioequivalent drug products must contain the same active ingredient in the same chemical form and in the same amount (i.e., they must be pharmaceutical equivalents), and they must have the same rate and extent of systemic drug absorption (i.e., the same bioavailability). The inactive ingredients or excipients may be different.

129. The answer is C (I, II).
Theophylline is an agent that is dependent on the cytochrome P-450 microsomal enzyme for its metabolism. Tobacco tars and phenobarbital are both considered to be enzyme inducers of the cytochrome P-450 microsomal enzyme system; consequently, theophylline metabolism may be increased in patients taking these agents concurrently. The H2-receptor antagonists cimetidine and ranitidine have both been shown to inhibit the P-450 enzyme system and thus reduce theophylline metabolism.

130. The answer is B.
Anemia is a common complication of chronic renal failure caused by a decrease in production of erythropoietin and endocrine product in the kidney. Erythropoietin, or epoetin alfa (Epogen, Procrit), stimulates red blood cell production in the bone marrow. This production is reflected by an increase in hematocrit and hemoglobin and a decrease in the need for blood transfusions. Recently, erythropoietin has been approved for the treatment of anemia in HIV-positive patients or for the prevention of anemia due to zidovudine (AZT).

131. The answer is C.
The most frequently reported adverse effects of raloxifene include hot flashes (up to 28% of women) and leg cramps (5.9%). Raloxifene has not been associated with irregular uterine bleeding or breast tenderness. Gastrointestinal complaints and allergic manifestations occur less frequently.

132. The answer is E (I, II, and III).
Emulsifying agents, also known as wetting agents, surfactants, or surface-active agents (e.g., soaps, sodium lauryl sulfate, and dioctyl sodium sulfosuccinate), lower the surface and interfacial tension. These agents permit more intimate contact between an aqueous (water) phase and a lipid phase.

133. The answer is B.
Ketoprofen is an NSAID structurally related to other propionic acids (ibuprofen, naproxen, fenoprofen). Indomethacin is an indoleacetic acid derivative; mefenamic acid is an anthranilic acid; aspirin is a salicylate; ketorolac is a pyrrolopyrrole.

134. The answer is E (I, II, and III).
Pyrimethamine, trimethoprim, and methotrexate act on the folic acid pathway to inhibit reduction of dihydrofolic acid to tetrahydrofolic acid by the enzyme dihydrofolate reductase.

135. The answer is D.
Salicylic acid is commonly used externally as a keratolytic in corn and wart preparations (e.g., Wart-Off and Freezone) to remove the horny layers of the skin in a process known as desquamation.

136. The answer is D.
Products containing benzoyl peroxide, sulfur, salicylic acid (3–6%), and resorcinol (1–2%) have been shown to be effective agents in the treatment of acne vulgaris. Benzoyl peroxide (Fostex), salicylic acid (PROPApH), sulfur (Liquimat and Fostex Medicated Cover-Up), and resorcinol and sulfur (Rezamid Lotion) are available OTC anti-acne products. Carmol-HC, a urea-containing product that also contains hydrocortisone, is effective in treating dry skin.

137. The answer is B (III).
Patients with type I, or insulin-dependent, diabetes are normally younger, are not obese, have an absolute lack of insulin in the pancreas, and are predisposed to ketoacidosis if they do not receive insulin.

138. The answer is B.
The choices are all steroids. Estrogenic steroids have an aromatic "A" ring. Progesterone and other progestins are derivatives of pregnane.

139. The answer is D.
Any disturbance in the balance between dopaminergic receptors and cholinergic receptors seems to result in various movement disorders. Increases in acetylcholine and decreases in dopamine, norepinephrine, serotonin, or gamma-aminobutyric acid (GABA) have all been linked to the development of various forms of Parkinson's disease. These alterations may occur because of the aging process, infection, drug consumption, or trauma.

140. The answer is B.
Aliphatic phenothiazine derivatives such as chlorpromazine and the piperidine derivatives mesoridazine (Serentil) and thioridazine (Mellaril) have the lowest risk for extrapyramidal side effects. Piperazine derivatives such as acetophenazine (Tindal), perphenazine (Trilafon), trifluoperazine (Stelazine), and fluphenazine (Prolixin), along with the thioxanthene derivatives thiothixene (Navane) and chlorprothixene (Taractan), have the highest likelihood of causing extrapyramidal side effects among the phenothiazines. The butyrophenone derivative haloperidol (Haldol) and the dihydroindolone derivative molindone (Moban) are also highly capable of inducing extrapyramidal side effects.

141. The answer is D.
Aminophylline, the parenteral form of theophylline, is commonly available as the dihydrate salt and contains approximately 80% theophylline. Enter this information into the calculation of the final serum

concentration by first converting the aminophylline dose into the equivalent theophylline dose. The expected serum concentration then can be calculated by dividing the corrected theophylline dose by the volume of distribution and adding that to the initial level of 7.5 mg/ml in this patient. The calculations are as follows:

$$250 \text{ mg aminophylline bolus} = 200 \text{ mg theophylline}$$
$$250 \times 0.80 = 200$$

$$C = \frac{\text{Dose}}{\text{Vd}} = \frac{200 \text{ mg}}{0.5 \text{ L/kg}} = \frac{200 \text{ mg}}{0.5 \text{ L/kg} \times 71.8 \text{ kg}} = \frac{200 \text{ mg}}{36 \text{ L}} = 5.55 \text{ μg/ml}$$

$$5.55 + 7.5 = 13.05 = 13.1 \text{ μg/ml}$$

142. The answer is E (I, II, and III).
Drugs that follow two-compartment pharmacokinetics have a rapid distribution phase, followed by a slower elimination phase representing the elimination of the drug after equilibration with the body. The plasma drug concentration at any time is the sum of two first-order processes. The slope of the terminal elimination phase, b, is generally used in the calculation of a dosage regimen.

143. The answer is D.
Competitive binding of cimetidine (and ranitidine) to the cytochrome P-450 mixed-function oxidase metabolic pathway of the liver acts to interfere with the metabolism of other drugs dependent on this pathway. Phenytoin, theophylline, phenobarbital, lidocaine, warfarin, imipramine, diazepam, and propranolol may be cleared more slowly and their effects may be accentuated if they are administered concomitantly with cimetidine or ranitidine.

144. The answer is D (II, III).
First-order elimination kinetics is expressed as $c = c_0 e^{-kt}$, where $c = 1.2$ mg/ml, $c_0 = 6.2$ mg/ml, and $t = 11$ h. By substitution, $1.2 = 6.2 e^{-k(11)}$. $k = 0.149$ h^{-1}. The $t_{1/2}$ is estimated by the relationship, $t_{1/2} = 0.693/k$. Therefore, $t_{1/2} = 0.693/0.149 = 4.65$ h. The dose and serum concentration must be known to determine the volume of distribution for this patient. A dose of 100 mg is reported to achieve a Cmax of 7.2 μg/ml based on a trough value of 1.2 μg/ml, or an increase of 6.0 μg/ml.

$$Vd = \frac{100 \text{ mg}}{6.0 \text{ μg/ml}} = 16.6 \text{ L, or } 0.23 \text{ L/kg}$$

145. The answer is D.
The minimum inhibitory concentration (MIC) for an antibiotic indicates the lowest concentration of antibiotic that prevents microbial growth after 18 to 24 hours of incubation. Typically, the peak antibiotic concentration at the site of infection must be four to five times the MIC to be considered therapeutic and effective.

146. The answer is B.
True cross-reactivity between cephalosporin antibiotics and penicillin is considered rare. Commonly, the rate of cross-reactivity is approximately 10%.

147. The answer is D.
If the patient is receiving 32 mg theophylline per hour by IV infusion, then the patient should receive the oral dose of theophylline at the same approximate dosing rate:
Theophylline dose = 32 mg ×12 h = 384 mg
Therefore, the patient should be given 400 mg of theophylline controlled-release product every 12 hours.

148. The answer is E (I, II, and III).
Conversion from IV to oral theophylline dosing should be accomplished using a sustained-release theophylline preparation designed to deliver a daily dose of theophylline comparable to the dose from the IV infusion. Although food may delay the achievement of a "peak" theophylline level, the amount absorbed is not compromised. A steady-state theophylline level is achievable if no doses are missed within the preceding 48-hour period. Reasonable sampling time should be within 3 to 7 hours of dosing.

149. The answer is C (I, II).
To demonstrate bioequivalency of two products, both must be the same dosage form (e.g., both must be controlled-release tablets), both must contain the same amount of the same active ingredient, and both must be given in the same dose and via the same route of administration. This manufacturer's study is, instead, a bioavailability study to demonstrate the controlled-release characteristics of the tablet.

150. The answer is C.
Combivent is a combination of ipratropium and albuterol.

151. The answer is C (I, II).
Dextromethorphan is a dextro-isomer of levorphanol, and many clinicians consider it equivalent to codeine as an antitussive. It depresses the cough center in the medulla. Diphenhydramine has both antitussive and antihistamine properties. Its antitussive effect results from direct medullary action. Dihydrocodeinone (hydrocodone) is a narcotic antitussive available only in prescription products.

152. The answer is E (I, II, and III).
Propylthiouracil (PTU) and methimazole may help attain remission in hyperthyroid patients. Both agents inhibit iodide oxidation and iodotyrosyl coupling. PTU (but not methimazole) also diminishes peripheral deiodination of thyroxine (T4) to triiodothyronine (T3). These drugs can be used to induce remission by themselves or as adjunctive therapy with radioiodine. They can be used for preoperative preparation of hyperthyroid patients to establish and maintain a euthyroid state until definitive surgery can be performed. Dermatologic reactions (e.g., rash, urticaria, pruritus, hair loss, and skin pigmentation) are the most troublesome. Patients receiving either PTU or methimazole are at increased risk for developing agranulocytosis.

153. The answer is B (III).
Atropine is a belladonna alkaloid that possesses anticholinergic properties. Vincristine (Oncovin) and vinblastine (Velban) are vinca alkaloids used in the treatment of various malignancies.

154. The answer is E.
Metronidazole is effective therapy for amebic dysentery, giardiasis, trichomoniasis, and infections caused by gram-negative anaerobes, including *Bacteroides fragilis.* It is not active against most aerobic gram-negative organisms, including *Escherichia coli.*

155. The answer is E (I, II, and III).
Ampules, the oldest form of parenteral vehicle, are composed entirely of glass, which may break during transport. Because the ampule is cut open on use, glass particles may be mixed with the drug substance. Therefore, all drugs supplied in ampules must be filtered before use to remove any glass particles from the solution. Once broken open, the solution must be used to avoid contamination, and it is therefore not a multiple-dose product.

156. The answer is B.
Half-normal saline solution (0.45% sodium chloride) has an osmotic pressure less than that of blood and is referred to as a hypotonic solution. Isotonic and isosmotic solutions have osmotic pressures that are equal to blood. Normal saline solution, 0.9% sodium chloride, usually is given as an example of an isotonic solution. Hypertonic solutions have osmotic pressures greater than blood (e.g., high concentrations of dextrose used in total parenteral therapy).

157. The answer is A (I).
Drug substances that have narrow therapeutic indexes (i.e., where the difference between a therapeutic effect and a toxic effect is small [e.g., heparin]) may be given via the continuous infusion route. This method allows less fluctuation in blood levels of such drugs. Intermittent infusions, although used extensively in medicine, provide for greater differences between peak effects and trough effects compared to agents with narrow therapeutic indexes. Agents such as norepinephrine, nitroprusside, and dopamine, which have very short half-lives, are routinely given by continuous infusion to provide a continuous therapeutic effect, which would not be available from intermittent dosing.

158. The answer is B.
Aluminum hydroxide (Amphojel) is used in patients with renal failure because it binds excess phosphate in the intestine, thereby reducing the serum phosphate concentration. The aluminum hydroxide can be in liquid or tablet form and is administered three or four times daily with meals.

159. The answer is A.
Kayexalate, or sodium polystyrene sulfonate (SPS), is an ion-exchange resin that exchanges sodium ion for potassium in the intestines. SPS, with its potassium content, is excreted in the feces. The result is a decrease in potassium levels in the serum and other body fluids.

160. The answer is A.
Chronic renal failure causes a normochromic, normocytic anemia, usually reflected in a decreased hemoglobin and decreased hematocrit. In most patients, the hematocrit is between 20% and 30%.

161. The answer is D (II, III).
The major route of elimination for both digoxin and tobramycin (an aminoglycoside) is the kidney. Both medications require dosage adjustment in patients with acute or chronic renal failure. Haloperidol is mainly metabolized by the liver and therefore would not need dosage adjustment.

162. The answer is C.
Calcitriol is 1,25-dihydroxycholecalciferol, the active form of vitamin D2. Because of its increased efficacy, calcitriol is the preferred form of vitamin D therapy used in patients with renal failure. Vitamin D enhances calcium absorption from the gut and is used to treat the hypocalcemia that occurs in renal failure.

163. The answer is C (I, II).
Aluminum hydroxide gel (Amphojel), which is used to treat the patient's hyperphosphatemia, and sodium polystyrene sulfonate (SPS) (Kayexalate), which is used to treat his hyperkalemia, are both major causes of constipation.

164. The answer is A (I).
IV calcium chloride or gluconate is used to treat potassium-induced arrhythmias. Loop diuretics and sodium polystyrene sulfonate (SPS) do not have a significant effect on potassium in a short period to treat life-threatening arrhythmia. SPS and loop diuretics, along with dialysis, may be considered to remove potassium in the short term, preventing recurrence of arrhythmias.

165. The answer is B.
The most common adverse reaction to haloperidol is extrapyramidal effects, which include dystonic reactions, akinesia, drug-induced parkinsonism, and tardive dyskinesia. Cardiovascular and anticholinergic side effects occur less frequently. Neuroleptic malignant syndrome is rare. A decreased seizure threshold is uncommon, except in patients with a history of seizures.

166. The answer is A (I).
Antacids, when given at the same time as cimetidine, decrease the absorption of cimetidine from the stomach. No interaction occurs between cimetidine and Colace or ferrous sulfate.

167. The answer is E.
Chemotherapeutic agents may cause dysfunction of many organ systems. Patients treated with daunorubicin, doxorubicin, and mitoxantrone are at greater risk for developing cardiotoxicity, ranging from electrocardiogram changes to cardiomyopathy. The risk is dose-related and cumulative. Total dose for daunorubicin should not exceed 550 mg/m^2.

168. The answer is B (III).
Alopecia occurs 1 to 2 weeks after treatment with most chemotherapeutic agents. Neither cytarabine nor daunorubicin causes renal dysfunction or peripheral neuropathy.

169. The answer is B.
When extravasation takes place, the needle is left in place and excess drug is drawn off with a syringe. A corticosteroid is injected to reduce local inflammation. Ice can also be applied. Sodium bicarbonate can be injected when the extravasation involves doxorubicin and other anthracyclines. Local anesthetics (e.g., potassium chloride) are not recommended and can cause local tissue damage.

170. The answer is C.
Ortho-Novum 1/50 contains 50 mg estrogen. When it is continuously administered, the monthly menstrual period will be suppressed. After chemotherapy, thrombocytopenia and neutropenia can occur, and Ms. Peterson will be at risk for increased bleeding due to thrombocytopenia.

171. The answer is C (I, II).
The chemotherapeutic agents used to treat Ms. Peterson cause myelosuppression, with attendant infection and bleeding, usually 10 to 14 days after chemotherapy. White blood cell lines, leukocytes and granulocytes, and also platelets are affected because of their shorter life span.

172. The answer is A.
Chemotherapeutic agents may be toxic to the pharmacist if handled improperly; therefore, many organizations have developed special guidelines. A vertical (rather than horizontal) laminar flow hood should be used to prevent airborne particles from contaminating room air. Special techniques, equipment, and protective gowns and gloves are recommended.

173. The answer is B.
Nystatin is an antifungal agent similar to amphotericin B. Its spectrum of activity includes *Histoplasma capsulatum* and *Candida albicans.* Nystatin suspension is used for treatment and prophylaxis of a common complication in immunocompromised cancer patients—oral thrush (*Candida*).

174. The answer is D.
Ms. Peterson is allergic to penicillin. Cross-sensitivity between cephalosporins and penicillins is currently approximately 10%. The literature still recommends caution when cephalosporins are administered to patients with acute nonlymphocytic leukemia and an allergy to penicillin.

175. The answer is B (III).
Gentamicin, an aminoglycoside, is excreted unchanged in the urine. The drug accumulates in the proximal tubule, causing renal damage in up to 25% of patients. The aminoglycosides do not cause hepatotoxicity or neurotoxicity.

176. The answer is D.
The approved dosage of ranitidine for management of gastroesophageal reflux disease (GERD) is 150 mg qid. GERD treatment requires aggressive acid inhibition that will maintain the esophageal pH at 4 or greater around the clock. Higher doses of ranitidine have not been proven to improve outcomes in GERD patients; lower doses may provide some improvement in heartburn symptoms but are less effective in eliminating symptoms or healing erosive esophagitis.

177. The answer is B.
Bleeding abnormalities result from vitamin K deficiency because of reduced formation of clotting factors II, VII, IX, and X.

178. The answer is B.
Body surface area correlates with cardiac output, which determines renal and hepatic blood flow and thus affects drug elimination.

179. The answer is B.
When weak acids are presented to the kidney for elimination, drugs that increase the ionization of these agents also increase their elimination. However, weak acids (e.g., methenamine) have their elimination delayed when agents such as aspirin decrease their ionization. This relative increase in un-ionized methenamine results in greater reabsorption of methenamine and, therefore, an increase in activity.

180. The answer is A.
Numerous hemorrhoid preparations are available OTC to treat the discomforts associated with hemorrhoids. These products contain steroids, astringents, anesthetics, and vasoconstrictors. However, Anusol-HC contains a local anesthetic combined with a concentration of hydrocortisone, which makes it a prescription item. Anusol is available OTC as a single-entity anesthetic product for the treatment of hemorrhoids. A low-strength form of Anusol-HC has been released OTC.

181. The answer is D.
Transdermal fentanyl is a controlled-release dosage form that is effective for a 72-hour period. All of the other drugs listed are effective for periods of 1–8 hours.

182. The answer is B.
Burow's solution is an aluminum acetate solution commonly used as an astringent solution and as an astringent mouthwash and gargle. Aluminum acetate is found in products that treat diaper rash, athlete's foot, and poison ivy.

183. The answer is E (I, II, and III).
Activase (recombinant tissue plasminogen activator) is a thrombolytic agent. Neupogen (granulocyte colony-stimulating factor [G-CSF]) is a cytokine that regulates the proliferation and differentiation of white blood cells. Epogen (recombinant erythropoietin) stimulates the production of red blood cells.

184. The answer is A (I).
Although anticholinergic agents have no proven value in ulcer healing, they have been used in conjunction with antacids for relief of refractory duodenal ulcer pain. An anticholinergic, Pro-Banthine (propantheline) can cause dry mouth, blurred vision, urinary retention, constipation, and pupillary dilation.

185. The answer is E (I, II, and III).
The liver is the main organ for the synthesis of plasma proteins. During end-stage liver disease, a decrease in plasma albumin concentrations leads to less drug protein binding and more free Coumadin drug concentrations, causing a more intense pharmacodynamic effect and therefore an increase in prothrombin time.

186. The answer is C.
To calculate the number of mEq KCl per tablet, divide the tablet strength (600 mg) by the mol wt (74.5). Each tablet contains 8 mEq KCl. The woman needs to take four tablets to provide a dose of 32 mEq KCl.

187. The answer is B.
The final suspension contains 8 g in 120 ml, which is 6.7% sucralfate (8/120 = 0.067 = 6.7%).

188. The answer is D.
The amount of sucralfate in 10 ml of this product is 0.667 g (8 g sucralfate/120 ml ×10 ml = 0.667 g sucralfate).

189. The answer is E (I, II, and III).
Passive diffusion follows Fick's principle of diffusion, in which the rate of diffusion is dependent on the concentration gradient, the partition coefficient (e.g., lipid solubility/water solubility ratio), and the surface area of the cell membrane. The extent of ionization relates the ratio of the nonionized or nonpolar species to the ionized or more water-soluble species.

190. The answer is B.
Psyllium is one of the bulk-forming laxatives. These agents absorb intestinal water and swell, increasing the bulk and moisture content of the stool to promote peristalsis. They act in both the small and large intestines.

PRESCRIPTION DISPENSING INFORMATION AND METROLOGY

Prescriptions

PARTS OF THE PRESCRIPTION

A prescription is an order for medication for use by a patient that is issued by a physician, dentist, veterinarian, or other licensed practitioner who is authorized to prescribe medication or by their agent via a collaborative practice agreement. A prescription is usually written on a single sheet of paper that is commonly imprinted with the prescriber's name, address, and telephone number. A medication order is similar to a prescription, but it is written on the patient chart and intended for use by a patient in an institutional setting.

All prescriptions should contain accurate and appropriate information about the patient and the medication that is being prescribed. In addition, a prescription order for a **controlled substance** must contain the following information:

1. Date of issue
2. Full name and address of the patient
3. Drug name, strength, dosage form, and quantity prescribed
4. Directions for use
5. Name, address, and Drug Enforcement Agency (DEA) number of the prescriber
6. Signature of the prescriber

A written prescription order is required for substances listed in **Schedule II.** Prescriptions for controlled substances listed in **Schedule II** are **never** refillable. Any other prescription that has no indication of refills is not refillable.

Prescriptions for medications that are listed in Schedules III, IV, and V may be issued either in writing or orally to the pharmacist. If authorized by the prescriber, these prescriptions may be refilled up to five times within 6 months of the date of issue. If the prescriber wishes the patient to continue to take the medication after 6 months or five refills, a new prescription order is required.

THE PRESCRIPTION LABEL

In addition to the name of the patient, the pharmacy, and the prescriber, the prescription label should accurately identify the medication and provide directions for its use.

The label for a prescription order for a controlled substance must contain the following information:

1. Name and address of the pharmacy
2. Serial number assigned to the prescription by the pharmacy
3. Date of the initial filling
4. Name of the patient
5. Name of the prescriber
6. Directions for use
7. Cautionary statements as required by law*

AUXILIARY LABELS

Auxiliary, or cautionary, labels provide additional important information about the proper use of the medication. Examples include "Shake Well" for suspensions or emulsions; "For External Use Only" for

---

*The label of any drug that is listed as a controlled substance in Schedule II, III, or IV of the Controlled Substances Act must contain the following warning: **CAUTION: Federal law prohibits the transfer of this drug to any person other than the patient for whom it was prescribed.**

topical lotions, solutions, or creams; and "May Cause Drowsiness" for medications that depress the central nervous system. The information contained on auxiliary labels should be brought to the attention of the patient when the medication is dispensed. The pharmacist should place only appropriate auxiliary labels on the prescription container because too many labels may confuse the patient.

BEFORE DISPENSING THE PRESCRIPTION

Double-check the accuracy of the prescription.
Provide undivided attention when filling the prescription.

1. Check the patient information (e.g., name, address, date of birth, telephone number).
2. Check the patient profile (e.g., allergies, medical conditions, other drugs, including over-the-counter medications).
3. Check the drug (e.g., correct drug name, correct spelling, appropriate drug for the patient's condition), and verify that there are no known drug interactions. **Always verify the name of the drug. Beware of drug names that look alike (see table).**
4. Check the dosage, including the drug strength, the dosage form (e.g., capsule, liquid, modified release), the individual dose, the total daily dose, the duration of treatment, and the units (e.g., mg, mL, tsp, tbsp).
5. Check the label. Compare the drug dispensed with the prescription. Verify the National Drug Code (NDC) number. Ensure that the information is accurate, that the patient directions are accurate and easily understood, and that the auxiliary labels are appropriate.
6. **Provide patient counseling. Be sure that the patient fully understands the drug treatment as well as any precautions.**

Examples of Drugs with Similar Names

Brand name	Celebrex	Cerebyx	Celexa
Generic name	Celecoxib capsules	Fosphenytoin sodium injection	Citalopram HCl
Manufacturer	Searle	Parke-Davis	Forest
Indication	Osteoarthritis and rheumatoid arthritis	Prevention and treatment of seizures	Major depression

Common Abbreviations

Considerable variation occurs in the use of capitalization, italicization, and punctuation in abbreviations. The following list shows the abbreviations that are most often encountered by pharmacists.

A, aa., or aa	of each	**mcg, mcg., or μg**	microgram
a.c.	before meals	**mEq**	milliequivalent
ad	to, up to	**mg or mg.**	milligram
a.d.	right ear	**ml or mL**	milliliter
ad lib.	at pleasure, freely	**μl or μL**	microliter
a.m.	morning	℔	minim
amp.	ampule	**N&V**	nausea and vomiting
ante	before	**Na**	sodium
aq.	water	**N.F.**	National Formulary
a.s.	left ear	**No.**	number
asa	aspirin	**noct.**	night, in the night
a.u.	each ear, both ears	**non rep.**	do not repeat
b.i.d.	twice a day	**NPO**	nothing by mouth
BP	British Pharmacopoeia	**N.S., NS, or N/S**	normal saline
BSA	body surface area	**1/2 NS**	half-strength normal saline
c. or c	with	**O**	pint
cap. or caps.	capsule	**o.d.**	right eye, every day
cp	chest pain	**o.l. or o.s.**	left eye
D.A.W.	dispense as written	**OTC**	over the counter
cc or cc.	cubic centimeter	**o.u.**	each eye, both eyes
comp.	compound, compounded	**oz.**	ounce
dil.	dilute	**p.c.**	after meals
D.C., dc, or disc.	discontinue	**PDR**	*Physicians' Desk Reference*
disp.	dispense	**p.m.**	afternoon, evening
div.	divide, to be divided	**p.o.**	by mouth
dl or dL	deciliter	**Ppt**	precipitated
d.t.d.	give of such doses	**pr**	for the rectum
DW	distilled water	**prn or p.r.n.**	as needed
D5W	dextrose 5% in water	**pt.**	pint
elix.	elixir	**pulv.**	powder
e.m.p.	as directed	**pv**	for vaginal use
et	and	**q.**	every
ex aq.	in water	**q.d.**	every day
fl or fld	fluid	**q.h.**	every hour
fl oz	fluid ounce	**q. 4 hr.**	every four hours
ft.	make	**q.i.d.**	four times a day
g or Gm	gram	**q.o.d.**	every other day
gal.	gallon	**q.s.**	a sufficient quantity
GI	gastrointestinal	**q.s. ad**	a sufficient quantity to make
gr or gr.	grain	**R**	rectal
gtt or gtt.	drop, drops	**R.L. or R/L**	Ringer's lactate
H	hypodermic	**℞**	prescription
h. or hr.	hour	**s. or s**	without
h.s.	at bedtime	**Sig.**	write on label
IM	intramuscular	**sol.**	solution
inj.	injection	**S.O.B.**	shortness of breath
IV	intravenous	**s.o.s.**	if there is need (once only)
IVP	intravenous push	**ss. or ss**	one-half
IVPB	intravenous piggyback	**stat.**	immediately
K	potassium	**subc, subq, or s.c.**	subcutaneously
l or L	liter	**sup. or supp**	suppository
lb.	pound	**susp.**	suspension
μ	Greek mu	**syr.**	syrup
M	mix	**tab.**	tablet
m² or M²	square meter	**tal.**	such, such a one

tal. dos.	such doses	**U or u.**	unit
tbsp. or T	tablespoonful	**u.d. or ut dict.**	as directed
t.i.d.	three times a day	**ung.**	ointment
tr. or tinct.	tincture	**U.S.P. or USP**	United States Pharmacopoeia
tsp. or t.	teaspoonful	**w/v**	weight/volume
TT	tablet triturates		

Metrology

THE METRIC, APOTHECARY, AND AVOIRDUPOIS SYSTEMS

Metric system

1. Basic units

Mass = g or gram
Length = m or meter
Volume = L or liter
1 cc (cubic centimeter) of water is approximately equal to 1 mL and weighs 1 g.

2. Prefixes

kilo- 10^3, or 1000 times the basic unit
hekto- 10^2, or 100 times the basic unit
deka-   10, or 10 times the basic unit
deci- 10^{-1}, or 0.1 times the basic unit
centi- 10^{-2}, or 0.01 times the basic unit
milli- 10^{-3}, or 0.001 times the basic unit
micro- 10^{-6}, or one-millionth of the basic unit
nano- 10^{-9}, or one-billionth of the basic unit
pico- 10^{-12}, or one-trillionth of the basic unit

Examples of these prefixes include milligram (mg), which equals one-thousandth of a gram, and deciliter (dl), which equals 100 mL, or 0.1 L.

Apothecary system

1. Volume (fluids or liquid)

60 minims (℔) = 1 fluidrachm or fluidram (f ʒ) or (ʒ)
8 fluidrachms (480 minims) = 1 fluidounce (f ℥ or ℥)
16 fluidounces = 1 pint (pt or 0)
2 pints (32 fluidounces) = 1 quart (qt)
4 quarts (8 pints) = 1 gallon (gal or C)

2. Mass (weight)

20 grains (gr) = 1 scruple (Э)
3 scruples (60 grains) = 1 drachm or dram (ʒ)
8 drachms (480 grains) = 1 ounce (℥)
12 ounces (5760 grains) = 1 pound (lb)

Avoirdupois system

1. Volume

1 fluidrachm = 60 min.
1 fluid ounce = 8 fl. dr.
              = 480 min.
1 pint = 16 fl. oz.
       = 7680 min.

```
1 quart  = 2 pt.
         = 32 fl. oz.
1 gallon = 4 qt.
         = 128 fl. oz.
```

2. Mass (weight)

The grain is common to both the apothecary and the avoirdupois systems.

437.5 grains (gr) = 1 ounce (oz)
16 ounces (7000 grains) = 1 pound (lb)

CONVERSION

Exact equivalents

Exact equivalents are used for the conversion of specific quantities in pharmaceutical formulas and prescription compounding.

1. Length

1 meter (m) = 39.37 in.
 1 inch (in) = 2.54 cm.

2. Volume

```
       1 ml = 16.23 minims (♏)
       1 ♏ = 0.06 mL
     1 f ʒ = 3.69 mL
     1 f ʒ = 29.57 mL
       1 pt = 473 mL
1 gal (U.S.) = 3785 mL
```

3. Mass

```
       1 g = 15.432 gr
      1 kg = 2.20 lb (avoir.)
      1 gr = 0.065 g or 65 mg
1 oz (avoir.) = 28.35 g
1 ʒ (apoth.) = 31.1 g
1 lb (avoir.) = 454 g
1 lb (apoth.) = 373.2 g
```

4. Other equivalents

```
 1 oz (avoir.) = 437.5 gr
 1 ʒ (apoth.) = 480 gr
 1 gal (U.S.) = 128 fl ʒ
1 fl ʒ (water) = 455 gr
 1 gr (apoth.) = 1 gr (avoir.)
```

Approximate equivalents

Physicians may use approximate equivalents to prescribe the dose quantities using the metric and apothecary systems of weights and measures, respectively. Household units are often used to inform the patient of the size of the dose. In view of the almost universal practice of using an ordinary household teaspoon to administer medication, a teaspoon may be considered 5 mL. However, when accurate measurement of a liquid dose is required, the USP recommends the use of a calibrated oral syringe or dropper.

```
1 fluid dram = 1 teaspoonful
             = 5 mL
4 fluidounces = 120 mL
8 fluidounces = 1 cup
             = 240 mL
   1 grain = 65 mg
      1 kg = 2.2 pounds (lb)
```

Surface Area Nomograms
Body Surface Area of Adults and Children[a]

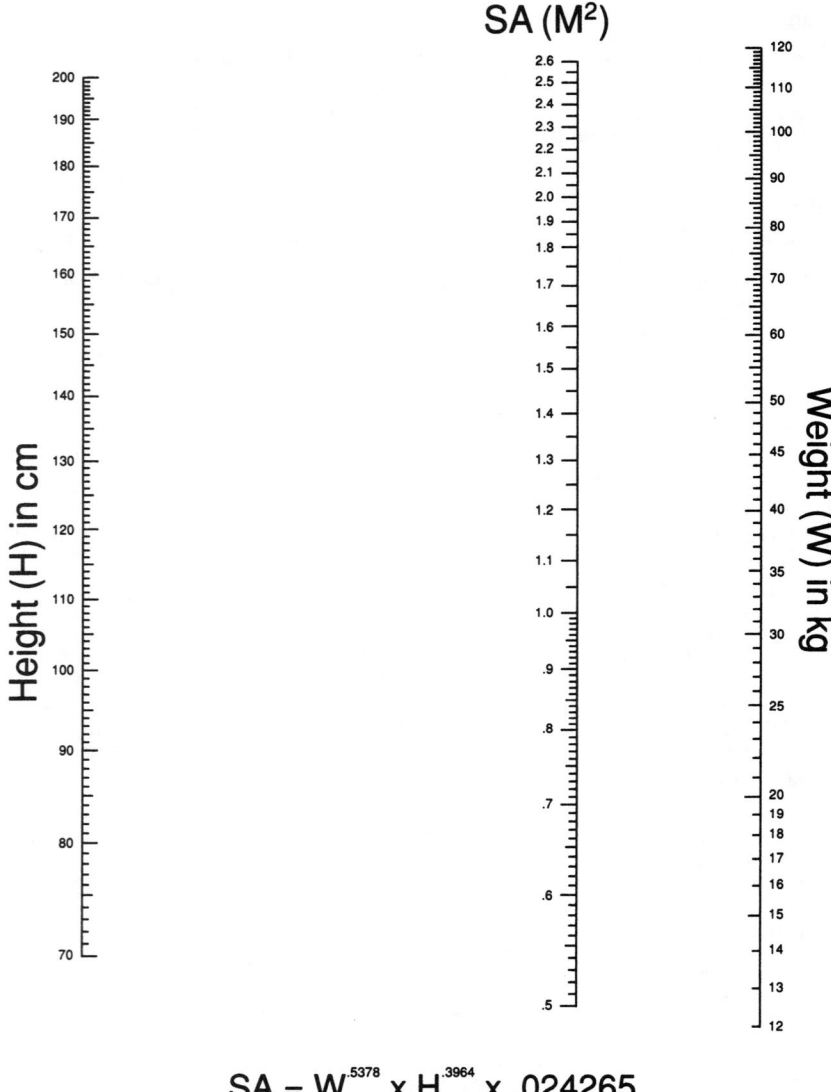

$$SA = W^{.5378} \times H^{.3964} \times .024265$$

Nomogram showing the relation among height, weight, and surface area in adults and children. To use the nomogram, align a ruler with the height and weight on the two lateral axes. The point at which the ruler intersects the center line shows the surface area. (Reprinted with permission from Haycock GB, Schwartz GJ, Wisotsky DH. Geometric method for measuring body surface area: a height–weight formula validated in infants, children, and adults. *J Pediatr* 1978;93:62–66.)

Body Surface Area of Infants*

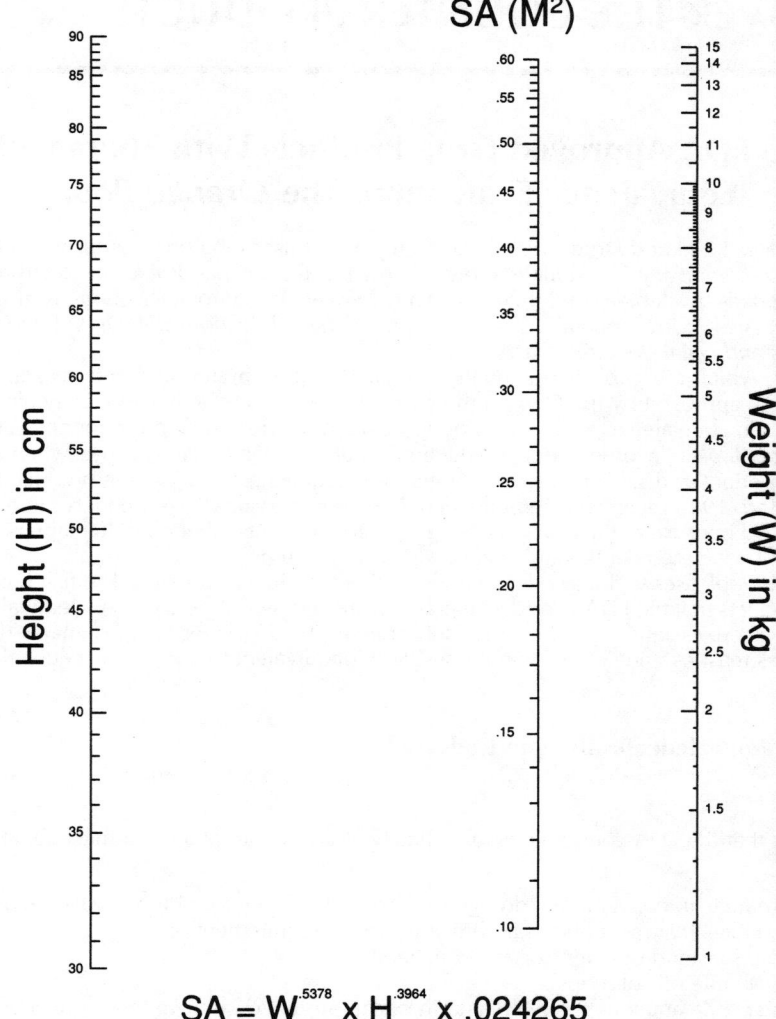

$$SA = W^{.5378} \times H^{.3964} \times .024265$$

Nomogram showing the relation among height, weight, and surface area in infants. To use the nomogram, align a ruler with the height and weight on the two lateral axes. The point at which the ruler intersects the center line shows the surface area. (Reprinted with permission from Haycock GB, Schwartz GJ, Wisotsky DH. Geometric method for measuring body surface area: a height–weight formula validated in infants, children, and adults. *J Pediatr* 1978;93: 62–66.)

COMMON PRESCRIPTION DRUGS AND OVER-THE-COUNTER PRODUCTS

The FDA Approved Drug Products With Therapeutic Equivalence Evaluation: The *Orange Book*

The United States Food and Drug Administration (FDA) publishes the book, *Approved Drug Products With Therapeutic Equivalence Evaluation,* often known as the *Orange Book.* An electronic version of the *Orange Book* is available on the Internet at http://www.fda/cder/ob. This book is also reproduced by the United States Pharmacopeial Convention, Inc., in the publication, USP DI, Volume III, *Approved Drug Products and Legal Requirements.*

These texts, which are published annually, identify the prescription and nonprescription products that are formally approved by the FDA on the basis of safety and effectiveness. They also provide the FDA's therapeutic equivalence evaluations for approved multiple-source prescription drug products.

The *Orange Book* is a drug product selection guide for pharmacists to use when dispensing a generic drug product as a substitute for the brand-name equivalent. A few drug products that were on the market before 1938 received a "grandfathered" FDA approval. These products are assumed to be safe and effective because of their long usage (e.g., digoxin tablets, phenobarbital tablets). These older products do not have therapeutic equivalence ratings at this time.

The *Orange Book* uses various codes to indicate therapeutic equivalence. The first letter "A" designates drug products that the FDA considers therapeutically equivalent to a pharmaceutically equivalent drug product. These products can be safely substituted. The first letter "B" designates drug products that, for various reasons, the FDA does not consider bioequivalent to the pharmaceutically equivalent drug product.

Therapeutic Equivalence Evaluation Codes

A Codes

Drug products that the FDA considers therapeutically equivalent to other pharmaceutically equivalent products

AA	Products in conventional dosage forms that do not present bioequivalence problems
AB	Products that meet necessary bioequivalence requirements
AN	Solutions and powders for aerosolization
AO	Injectable oil solutions
AP	Injectable aqueous solutions, and in certain instances, intravenous nonaqueous solutions
AT	Topical products

B Codes

Drug products that the FDA does not consider therapeutically equivalent to other pharmaceutically equivalent products at this time

B*	Drug products that require further FDA investigation and review to determine therapeutic equivalence
BC	Extended-release dosage forms (capsules, injectables, and tablets)
BD	Active ingredients and dosage forms that have documented problems with bioequivalence
BE	Delayed-release oral dosage forms
BN	Products in aerosol–nebulizer drug-delivery systems
BP	Active ingredients and dosage forms that have potential problems with bioequivalence
BR	Suppositories or enemas that deliver drugs for systemic absorption
BS	Drug products that have drug standard deficiencies
BT	Topical products that have bioequivalence issues
BX	Drug products for which the data are insufficient to determine therapeutic equivalence

Drug Class Symbols

The following symbols indicate the drug class of products under the Controlled Substances Act of 1970. They apply to all drug products in which they appear. These symbols are intended for use only as a guide. Check the manufacturer's label for definitive information.

C-I Drug substances that have a high potential for abuse and have no accepted medical use in the United States. Examples include heroin, peyote, LSD, mescaline, and psilocybin.

C-II Drug substances that have a high potential for abuse, but have a currently acceptable medical use in drug treatment. Prescriptions must be written in ink or typewritten and signed by the practitioner. Verbal prescriptions must be confirmed in writing within 72 hours and may be given only in a genuine emergency. No renewals are permitted. Examples include morphine, amphetamines, and barbiturates.

C-III Drug substances that have some potential for abuse. Prescriptions may be oral or written. Up to 5 renewals are permitted in 6 months.

C-IV Drug substances that have a low potential for abuse. Prescriptions may be oral or written. Up to 5 renewals are permitted in 6 months.

C-V Drug substances that are subject to state and local regulation. The potential for abuse is low. A prescription may be required.

Rx Drug substances that are available by prescription only, but are not classified as controlled substances.

Top 200 Prescription Drugs by Trade Name

The following list contains the top 200 brand-name prescription drugs dispensed through independent, chain, food store, mass merchandiser, and deep discount pharmacies. Rankings are based on total number of prescriptions for January to December 2001, as measured by Scott-Levin's Source Prescription Audit. Insulin products are included in the tally.

Rank	Product	Rank	Product
1	Lipitor	29	Accupril
2	Synthroid	30	Pravachol
3	Premarin Tabs	31	Neurontin
4	Norvasc	32	Lanoxin
5	Prilosec	33	Wellbutrin SR
6	Zoloft	34	Prinivil
7	Zithromax Z-Pak	35	Ultram
8	Claritin	36	Flonase
9	Paxil	37	Singulair
10	Celebrex	38	Glucotrol XL
11	Glucophage	39	Coumadin Tabs
12	Prevacid	40	Levaquin
13	Vioxx	41	Amoxil
14	Augmentin	42	Effexor XR
15	Zocor	43	Diflucan
16	Zestril	44	Flovent
17	Ortho Tri-Cyclen	45	Lotensin
18	Prempro	46	Nasonex
19	Levoxyl	47	Zithromax, Oral Suspension
20	Allegra	48	Plavix
21	Ambien	49	K-Dur 20
22	Zyrtec	50	Lotrel
23	Prozac	51	Cozaar
24	Celexa	52	Avandia
25	Toprol XL	53	Depakote
26	Viagra	54	Claritin D, 24-hr.
27	Fosamax	55	Diovan
28	Cipro	56	Risperdal

(Continued on next page)

Rank	Product	Rank	Product
57	Claritin D, 12-hr.	116	Miacalcin Nasal
58	Adderall	117	Nasacort AQ
59	Humulin N	118	Detrol
60	Xalatan	119	Endocet
61	Allegra-D	120	Biaxin XL
62	Oxycontin	121	Tequin
63	Klor-Con	122	Loestrin Fe 1/20
64	Altace	123	Relafen
65	Actos	124	Tobradex
66	Serevent	125	Seroquel
67	Zyprexa	126	Humalog
68	Evista	127	Atrovent Inhalation
69	Monopril	128	Phenergan Suppositories
70	Aciphex	129	Adalat CC
71	Protonix	130	Proventil HFA
72	Veetids	131	Tussionex
73	Hyzaar	132	Loestrin Fe 1.5/30
74	Amaryl	133	Aricept
75	Combivent	134	Alphagan
76	Flomax	135	Zithromax
77	Ortho-Novum 7/7/7	136	Lo/Ovral 28
78	Cefzil	137	Patanol
79	Levothroid	138	Coreg
80	Dilantin Kapseals	139	Apri
81	Zestoretic	140	Lotrisone
82	Ceftin	141	Azmacort
83	Alesse-28	142	Rhinocort Aqua
84	Roxicet	143	Ditropan XL
85	Diovan HCT	144	Pepcid
86	Ortho-Cyclen	145	Differin
87	Biaxin	146	Low-Ogestrel
88	Imitrex Oral	147	Atacand
89	Humulin 70/30	148	Prinzide
90	Serzone	149	Climara
91	Valtrex	150	Demadex
92	Macrobid	151	Ciloxan
93	Digitek	152	Estratest Tabs
94	Concerta	153	Humulin R
95	Necon 1/35	154	Benzamycin
96	Claritin RediTabs	155	Duragesic
97	Glucovance	156	Lamisil Oral
98	Baycol	157	Topamax
99	Avapro	158	Cardizem CD
100	Bactroban	159	Guaifenex PSE
101	Glucophage XR	160	Proscar
102	Triphasil	161	Omnicef
103	Mircette	162	Zanaflex
104	Skelaxin	163	Prometrium
105	Lescol	164	Mobic
106	Zyrtec Syrup	165	Vasotec
107	Remeron	166	Desogen
108	Nexium	167	Ocuflox
109	Tricor	168	Premphase
110	Tiazac	169	Xenical
111	Plendil	170	Niaspan
112	Trivora-28	171	Estratest HS
113	Advair Diskus	172	Estrostep Fe
114	Elocon	173	MetroGel Vaginal
115	Vicoprofen, Non-Injectable	174	Detrol LA

Rank	Product	Rank	Product
175	Accolate	188	Zaroxolyn
176	Actonel	189	Sonata
177	Univasc	190	Cosopt
178	Procardia XL	191	Axid
179	Covera-HS	192	Nizoral Shampoo
180	Zantac	193	Zovia 1/35
181	Lac-Hydrin	194	Terazol 7
182	Thyroid, Armour	195	Avelox
183	Asacol	196	Avalide
184	Lotensin HCT	197	Rhinocort
185	Claritin Syrup	198	Xanax
186	Cardura	199	Accutane
187	Femhrt	200	Meridia

Source: Scott-Levin's Source Prescription Audit (SPA).

Reprinted with permission from *The Drug Topics Red Book*, Thomson Medical Economics: Montvale, NJ, 2002.

Top 200 Prescription Drugs by Generic Name

The following list contains the top 200 generic prescription drugs dispensed through independent, chain, food store, mass merchandiser, and deep discount pharmacies. Rankings are based on total number of prescriptions for January to December 2001, as measured by Scott-Levin's Source Prescription Audit.

Rank	Product	Rank	Product
1	Hydrocodone/APAP	33	Isosorbide Mononitrate
2	Atenolol	34	Albuterol Nebulizer Solution
3	Amoxicillin	35	Methylprednisone Tablets
4	Furosemide Oral	36	Allopurinol
5	Albuterol Aerosol	37	Estradiol Oral
6	Alprazolam	38	Clonidine
7	Hydrochlorothiazide	39	Fluoxetine
8	Propoxyphene-N/APAP	40	Penicillin VK
9	Cephalexin	41	Doxazosin
10	Triamterene w/HCTZ	42	Folic Acid
11	Ibuprofen	43	Temazepam
12	Acetaminophen w/Codeine	44	Oxycodone w/APAP
13	Prednisone Oral	45	Hydroxyzine
14	Trimox	46	Meclizine HCl
15	Lorazepam	47	Metronidazole Tablets
16	Metoprolol Tartrate	48	Gemfibrozil
17	Amitriptyline	49	Promethazine Tablets
18	Ranitidine HCl	50	Terazosin
19	Trimethoprim/Sulfate	51	Triamcinolone Acetonide Topical
20	Naproxen	52	Cartia XT
21	Cyclobenzaprine	53	Spironolactone
22	Clonazepam	54	Metoclopramide
23	Trazodone HCl	55	Minocycline
24	Diazepam	56	Bisoprolol/HCTZ
25	Verapamil SR	57	Nifedipine ER
26	Glyburide	58	Propranolol HCl
27	Enalapril	59	Promethazine/Codeine
28	Potassium Chloride	60	Acyclovir
29	Carisoprodol	61	Glipizide
30	Doxycycline	62	Captopril
31	Warfarin	63	Butalbital/APAP/Caffeine
32	Medroxyprogesterone Tablets		*(Continued on next page)*

Rank	Product	Rank	Product
64	Clindamycin Systemic	121	Nystatin/Triamcinolone
65	Diltiazem CD	122	Phenytoin Sodium Extended
66	Nortriptyline	123	Ibuprofen Liquid
67	Tamoxifen	124	Guaifenesin Rx
68	Methylphenidate	125	Diphenoxylate w/Atropine
69	Tetracycline	126	Isosorbide Dinitrate
70	Albuterol Oral Liquid	127	Diphenhydramine Tablets
71	Cimetidine	128	Colchicine
72	Benzonatate	129	Promethazine DM
73	Phenobarbital	130	Docusate Sodium
74	Naproxen Sodium	131	Cefactor
75	Nitroglycerin	132	Hydroxyzine Pamoate
76	Phenazopyridine HCl	133	Pentoxifylline
77	Ferrous Sulfate	134	Labetalol
78	Aspirin, Enteric-Coated	135	Estropipate
79	Hyoscyamine	136	Carbidopa/Levodopa
80	Guaifenesin/Pseudoephedrine	137	Baclofen
81	Buspirone HCl	138	Ketoconazole Topical
82	Quinine Sulfate	139	Gentamicin Ophthalmic
83	Phentermine	140	Amiodarone
84	Methocarbamol	141	Dexamethasone Oral
85	Propranolol LA	142	Glyburide Micronized
86	Diclofenac Sodium	143	Prednisolone Acetate
87	Dicyclomine HCl		Ophthalmic
88	Nitroquick	144	Clorazepate Dipotassium
89	Doxepin	145	Erythromycin Ophthalmic
90	Carbamazepine	146	Bumetanide, Non-Injectable
91	Famotidine	147	Polymyxin B/Trimethoprim
92	Ery-Tab	148	Cardec DM
93	Indomethacin	149	Nitrofurantoin Macrocrystals
94	Methotrexate	150	Ipratropium Bromide
95	Nystatin Systemic	151	Sodium Fluoride
96	Indapamide	152	Guaifenesin LA
97	Hydrocortisone Topical Rx	153	Quintex PSE
98	Imipramine HCl	154	Clotrimazole/Betamethasone
99	Diltiazem SR	155	Timolol Maleate GFS
100	Neomycin/Polymyxin/HC	156	Tobramycin Ophthalmic
101	Guiatuss AC	157	Haloperidol
102	Acetaminophen	158	Cefadroxil
103	Theophylline SR	159	Sulfatrim Pediatric
104	Prednisolone Oral	160	Hydrocortisone Valerate
105	Digoxin	161	Erythromycin Ethylsuccinate
106	Benztropine	162	Octicair
107	Prochlorperazine Maleate	163	Piroxicam
108	Atenolol Chlorthalidone	164	Timolol Maleate Ophthalmic
109	Chlorhexidine Gluconate	165	Clotrimazole Topical
110	Levothyroxine	166	Nifedipine
111	Hydroxychloroquine	167	Chlordiazepoxide w/Clidinium
112	Fluocinonide	168	Chlordiazepoxide HCl
113	Nadolol	169	HycoClear Tuss
114	Nystatin Topical	170	Prenatal Plus
115	Etodolac	171	Promethazine VC w/Codeine
116	Lithium Carbonate	172	Butalbital Compound
117	Oxybutynin Chloride	173	Triazolam
118	Clobetasol	174	Bupropion
119	Clindamycin Topical	175	Hydralazine
120	Multivitamins w/Fluoride,	176	Nifedical XL
	Chewable	177	Cyproheptadine

Rank	Product	Rank	Product
178	Erythromycin Topical	190	Guanfacine HCl
179	Tretinoin	191	Ketorolac Oral
180	Erythromycin Base	192	Lactulose
181	Orphenadrine Citrate	193	Lindane
182	Dipyridamole	194	Sulfasalazine
183	Sulindac	195	Methadone HCl, Non-Injectable
184	Butalbital Compound w/Codeine	196	Azathioprine
185	Phenobarbital/Belladonna	197	Promethazine VC
186	Morphine Sulfate, Non-Injectable	198	Enulose
187	Promethazine Liquid	199	Hemorrhoidal HC
188	Theochron	200	Cheratussin AC
189	Lonox		

Source: Scott-Levin's Source Prescription Audit (SPA).

Reprinted with permission from *The Drug Topics Red Book*, Thomson Medical Economics: Montvale, NJ, 2002.

Top OTC Drugs

The following list contains the Top OTC drugs by pharmacist recommendation in specific therapeutic classes.

Trade Name	Generic
Abreva	docosanol
Actifed	pseudoephedrine HCl (PSE), triprolidine HCl, acetaminophen (APAP)
Advil	ibuprofen
Afrin	oxymetazoline HCl
Aleve	naproxen sodium
ALternaGEL	aluminum hydroxide
Anusol	various formulations
Azo Standard	phenazopyridine hydrochloride
Bayer Aspirin	acetylsalicylic acid (ASA, aspirin)
Ben-Gay	methyl salicylate, menthol, and camphor
Benadryl Oral	diphenhydramine HCl (DPH), pseudoephedrine HCl (PSE), acetaminophen (APAP)
Betadine	povidine-iodine
Bonine	meclizine HCl
Bufferin	acetylsalicylic acid (ASA, aspirin) with buffers
Caladryl	pramoxine HCl, camphor with calamine or zinc acetate
Calcium	
Campho-Phenique	camphor, phenol, bacitracin zinc, neomycin sulfate, polymyxin B sulfate, lidocaine
Cepastat	phenol
Chlor-Trimeton	chlorpheniramine maleate (CPH), pseudoephedrine sulfate (PSE)
Chloraseptic	benzocaine and menthol or phenol
Citrucel	methylcellulose
Colace	docusate sodium
Compound W	salicylic acid
Comtrex	pseudoephedrine HCl (PSE), chlorpheniramine maleate (CPH), dextromethorphan HBr (DXT), acetaminophen (APAP), guaifenesin (GUA)
Contac	pseudoephedrine HCl (PSE), chlorpheniramine maleate (CPH), dextromethorphan HBr (DXT), acetaminophen (APAP), diphenhydramine HCl
Cortaid	hydrocortisone
Debrox	
Delsym	dextromethorphan polistirex
Dramamine and Dramamine II	dimenhydrinate or meclizine HCl

(Continued on next page)

Trade Name	Generic
Drixoral	pseudoephedrine sulfate (PSE), dexbrompheniramine maleate (DXB), acetaminophen (APAP)
Dulcolax	bisacodyl
Duofilm	salicylic acid
Emetrol	phosphorated carbohydrates
Excedrin	acetaminophen, aspirin, caffeine, diphenhydramine citrate
Femstat 3	butoconazole nitrate
FiberCon	polycarbophil calcium
Gas-X	simethicone, calcium carbonate
Gaviscon	aluminum hydroxide, magnesium trisilicate
Gyne-Lotrimin	clotrimazole
Imodium A-D	loperamide HCl
Kank-A	benzocaine, cetylpyridinium chloride
Kaopectate	bismuth subsalicylate
Lactinex	lactobacillus
Lamisil AT	terbinafine hydrochloride
Listerine	thymol, eucalyptol, methyl salicylate, and menthol
Lotrimin AF	clotrimazole or miconazole nitrate
Maalox/Maalox Plus	aluminum hydroxide, magnesium hydroxide, calcium carbonate, magnesium carbonate, simethicone
Metamucil	psyllium hydrophilic mucilloid
Midol/Midol PMS	pamabrom, pyrilamine maleate, acetaminophen, caffeine, ibuprofen
Monistat Vaginal	miconazole nitrate, tioconazole
Motrin IB	ibuprofen
Mylanta	aluminum hydroxide, magnesium (hydroxide and carbonate), calcium carbonate, simethicone
Mylanta Gas	simethicone
Mylicon Drops	simethicone
Myoflex	trolamine salicylate
Naphcon A	pheniramine maleate, naphazoline HCl
Nasalcrom	cromolyn sodium
Neo-Synephrine	phenylephrine HCl or oxymetazoline HCl
Neosporin	polymyxin B sulfate, neomycin, bacitracin, pramoxine HCl
Nicoderm CQ	nicotine Transdermal
Nicorette	nicotine Polacrilex
Nix	permethrin
Nizoral Shampoo	ketoconazole
NoDoz	caffeine
NyQuil	pseudoephedrine HCl (PSE), chlorpheniramine maleate (CPH), dextromethorphan HBr (DXT), acetaminophen (APAP), doxylamine succinate
Ocean	sodium chloride
Opcon A	pheniramine maleate, naphazoline HCl
OralBalance	glucose oxidase, lactoperoxidase, lysozyme
Orudis KT	ketoprofen
Pamprin	pamabrom, pyrilamine maleate, acetaminophen, magnesium salicylate
Pedia Care	pseudoephedrine HCl (PSE), chlorpheniramine maleate (CPH), dextromethorphan HBr (DXT)
Pepcid-AC	famotidine
Pepcid Complete	famotidine, calcium carbonate, magnesium hydroxide
Pepto Bismol	bismuth subsalicylate
Peri-Colace	docusate sodium and casanthranol
Phillips' MOM	magnesium hydroxide
Pin-X	pyrantel pamoate
Preparation H	shark liver oil, petrolatum, mineral oil, phenylephrine HCl
Primatine	epinephrine, ephedrine, guaifenesin
RID	pyrethrins

Trade Name	Generic
Robitussin (Adult)	guaifenesin (GUA)
Rogaine	minoxidil
Senokot	standardized senna concentrate with or without docusate
Sinutab	pseudoephedrine HCl (PSE), acetaminophen (APAP), chlorpheniramine maleate (CPH), guaifenesin
Sominex	diphenhydramine HCl
Sucrets	hexylresorcinol, dyclonine HCl, or dextromethorphan HBr
Sudafed	pseudoephedrine HCl (PSE), dextromethorphan HBr (DXT), acetaminophen (APAP), chlorpheniramine HCl (CPH), guaifenesin (GUA)
Tagamet HB 200	cimetidine
Tums	calcium carbonate
Tavist	clemastine fumarate, pseudoephedrine HCl, acetaminophen
Tears Naturale	hydroxypropyl methylcellulose, Dextran 70, white petrolatum, mineral oil
TheraFlu	pseudoephedrine HCl (PSE), chlorpheniramine maleate (CPH), acetaminophen (APAP), dextromethorphan HBr (DXT)
Tinactin	tolnaftate
Triaminic Oral	chlorpheniramine maleate (CPH), pseudoephedrine HCl (PSE) dextromethorphan HBr (DXT), guaifenesin (GUA) All formulations are alcohol-free.
Tylenol	acetaminophen (APAP)
Tylenol Allergy & Sinus	pseudoephedrine HCl (PSE), chlorpheniramine maleate (CPH), acetaminophen (APAP), doxylamine succinate
Tylenol Cold and Flu (Adult)	pseudoephedrine HCl (PSE), chlorpheniramine maleate (CPH), dextromethorphan HBr (DXT), acetaminophen (APAP), doxylamine succinate
Unisom	doxylamine succinate or diphenhydramine HCl
Visine	tetrahydrozoline HCl, oxymetazoline HCl, naphazoline HCl, pheniramine maleate
Vitamin A	retinol, retinoic acid, beta carotene, retinal, retinaldehyde; retinyl esters are all in the vitamin A family
Vitamin B Complex	vitamins B1 (thiamine), B2 (riboflavin), B3 (niacin), B5 (pantothenic acid), B6 (pyridoxine), B12 (cyanocobolamin), biotin, choline, folic acid, inositol, para-aminobenzoic acid
Vitamin C	ascorbic acid
Vitamin E	alpha-tocopherol
Zantac 75	ranitidine hydrochloride
Zostrix	capsaicin

Used with permission from *Nonprescription Drug Cards*. 4th ed. Sigler and Flanders, 2003.

APPENDIX C

REFERENCE CHARTS FOR PATIENT COUNSELING

Drugs That Should Not Be Crushed

Pharmacists may frequently encounter patients who, for one reason or another, cannot swallow tablets or capsules. When an alternative liquid formulation is not available, pulverizing the solid dosage form before administration may serve as a quick, safe solution to the problem.

However, not all pharmaceutical products may be crushed before administration. A variety of slow-release formulations can deliver dangerous immediate doses of their active ingredients if the integrity of the delivery system is destroyed, and enteric-coated products must remain intact in order to prevent their dissolution in the stomach.

Listed below are various slow-release as well as enteric-coated products which should not be crushed or chewed. Slow-release (sr) represents products that are controlled-release, extended-release, long-acting, and timed-release. Enteric-coated (ec) represents products that are delayed-release.

In general, capsules containing slow-release or enteric-coated particles may be opened and their contents administered on a spoonful of soft food. Instruct patients not to chew the particles, though. (Patients should, in fact, be discouraged from chewing any medication unless it is specifically formulated for that purpose.)

This list should be not considered all-inclusive. Generic and alternate brands of some products may exist. Tablets intended for sublingual or buccal administration (not included in this list) should also be administered only as intended, in an intact form.

Drug	Type of Release[a]	Drug	Type of Release
Abletex PSE	sr	Aquatab C	sr
Accuhist LA	sr	Aquatab D	sr
Aciphex	ec	Aquatab DM	sr
Adalat CC	sr	Aquatab-D	sr
Adderall XR	sr	Dose Pack	
Aerolate III	sr	Arthrotec	ec
Aerolate Jr	sr	Asacol	ec
Aerolate SR	sr	Ascocid-1000	sr
Aggrenox	sr	Ascocid-500-D	sr
Aleve Cold	sr	Ascriptin Enteric	ec
& Sinus		ATP	ec
Aleve Sinus &	sr	Atrohist	sr
Headache		Pediatric	
Allegra-D	sr	Azulfidine	ec
Allerx	sr	Entabs	
Allerx-D	sr	Bayer 8-Hour	sr
Allfen	sr	Extended	
Allfen-DM	sr	Release	
Alophen	ec	Bayer Arthritis	ec
Alterra	sr	Pain Regimen	
Amfed TD	sr	Bayer Aspirin	ec
Amibid DM	sr	Regimen	
Amibid LA	sr	Biaxin XL	sr
Amidal	sr	Bidex	sr
Aminoxin	ec	Bidex-DM	sr
Ami-Tex PSE	sr	Biohist LA	sr
Anatuss LA	sr	Bisac-Evac	ec
Aquabid-DM	sr	Biscolax	ec

Drug	Type of Release	Drug	Type of Release
Boca-Tex PSE	sr	Depakote	ec
Bontril Slow-Release	sr	Depakote ER	sr
		Depakote Sprinkles	ec
Bromadrine TR	sr		
Bromfed	sr	Desal II	sr
Bromfed-PD	sr	Despec SR	sr
Bromfenex	sr	Detrol LA	sr
Bromfenex PD	sr	Dexaphen SA	sr
Bufferin Low Dose	ec	Dexatrim	sr
		Dexedrine Spansules	sr
Caffedrine	sr		
Calan SR	sr	D-Feda II	sr
Carbatrol	sr	Diamox Sequels	sr
Cardene SR	sr	Dilacor XR	sr
Cardizem CD	sr	Dilantin Kapseals	sr
Cardizem SR	sr		
Carox Plus	sr	Dilatrate-SR	sr
Cartia XT	sr	Diltia XT	sr
Catemine	ec	Dimetane Extentabs	sr
Ceclor CD	sr		
Ceclor CDpak	sr	Disophrol Chronotab	sr
Cemill 1000	sr		
Cemill 500	sr	Ditropan XL	sr
Cevi-Bid	sr	Donnatal Extentabs	sr
Chlor-Phen	sr		
Chlor-Trimeton Allergy	sr	Doryx	ec
		Drexophed SR	sr
Chlor-Trimeton Allergy Decongestant Tablets	sr	Drituss GP	sr
		Drixomed	sr
		Drixoral	sr
		Drixoral Plus	sr
Choledyl SA	sr	Drixoral Sinus	sr
Claritin-D	sr	Drize-R	sr
Claritin-D 24 Hour	sr	Drysec	sr
		Dulcolax	ec
Coldec TR	sr	Duradryl Jr	sr
Compazine Spansule	sr	Durasal II	sr
		Duratuss	sr
Concerta	sr	Duratuss G	sr
Correctol	ec	Duratuss GP	sr
Cotazym-S	ec	Dura-Vent/DA	sr
Covera-HS	sr	Dylaxol	ec
Creon 10	ec	Dynabac	ec
Creon 20	ec	Dynabac D5-Pak	ec
Creon 5	ec	Dynacirc CR	sr
C-Tym	sr	Dynahist-ER Pediatric	sr
Cystospaz-M	sr		
D.A. II	sr	Dynex	sr
Dairycare	ec	Easprin	ec
Dallergy	sr	EC Naprosyn	ec
Dallergy Jr	sr	Ecotrin	ec
D-Amine-SR	sr		
Deconamine SR	sr	Ecotrin Adult Low Strength	ec
Decongest II	sr		
De-Congestine	sr	Ecotrin Maximum Strength	ec
Deconomed SR	sr		
Deconsal II	sr		
Defen-LA	sr		

(Continued on next page)

Drug	Type of Release	Drug	Type of Release
Ecpirin	ec	Guaimax-D	sr
Ed A-Hist	sr	Guaipax PSE	sr
Ed K+10	sr	Guai-Vent/PSE	sr
Effexor-XR	sr	Gua-SR	sr
Efidac 24 Chlorpheniramine	sr	Guiadrine DM	sr
		Guiadrine G-1200	sr
Efidac 24 Pseudoephedrine	sr	Guiadrine GP	sr
Empro	sr	Guiadrine PSE	sr
Endal	sr	Guiatex II SR	sr
Entercote	ec	Guiatex PSE	sr
Entex LA	sr	H 9600 SR	sr
Entex PSE	sr	Halfprin	ec
Entocort EC	ec	Histade	sr
Eryc	ec	Hista-Vent DA	sr
Ery-Tab	ec	Histex CT	sr
Eskalith-CR	sr	Histex SR	sr
Eudal SR	sr	Humavent LA	sr
Extendryl Jr	sr	Humibid DM	sr
Extendryl SR	sr	Humibid LA	sr
Extress-60	sr	Humibid Pediatric	sr
Feen-A-Mint	ec		
Femilax	ec	Iberet-500	sr
Femitrol	ec	Iberet-Folic-500	sr
Fenesin	sr	Icaps TR	sr
Fenesin DM	sr	Imdur	sr
Fero-Folic 500	sr	Inderal LA	sr
Fero-Grad-500	sr	Indocin SR	sr
Ferro-Sequels	sr	Iobid DM	sr
Ferro-Time	sr	Iofed	sr
Ferrous Fumarate DS	sr	Iofed PD	sr
		Ionamin	sr
Fetrin	sr	Iosal II	sr
Flagyl ER	sr	Iotex PSE	sr
Fleet Bisacodyl	ec	Isoptin SR	sr
Folitab 500	sr	K-10	sr
Fumatinic	sr	K-8	sr
Genacote	ec	Kadian	sr
GFN/PSE	sr	Kaon-Cl 10	sr
Giltuss TR	sr	K-Dur 10	sr
Glucophage XR	sr	K-Dur 20	sr
Glucotrol XL	sr	Klor-Con 10	sr
GP 500	sr	Klor-Con 8	sr
G-Phed	sr	Klor-Con M10	sr
G-Phed-PD	sr	Klor-Con M20	sr
Guaifed	sr	Klotrix	sr
Guaifed-PD	sr	Kronofed-A	sr
Guaifenex DM	sr	Kronofed-A-JR	sr
Guaifenex G	sr	K-Tab	sr
Guaifenex GP	sr	Lescol XL	sr
Guaifenex LA	sr	Levbid	sr
Guaifenex PSE 120	sr	Levsinex	sr
		Lexxel	sr
Guaifenex PSE 60	sr	Lipram 4500	ec
		Lipram-CR10	ec
Guaifenex-Rx	sr	Lipram-CR20	ec
Guaifenex-Rx DM	sr		

Drug	Type of Release	Drug	Type of Release
Lipram-PN10	ec	Norpace CR	sr
Lipram-PN16	ec	Omnihist L.A.	sr
Lipram-PN20	ec	Oramorph SR	sr
Lipram-UL12	ec	Oruvail	sr
Lipram-UL18	ec	Oxycontin	sr
Lipram-UL20	ec	Palgic-D	sr
Liquibid	sr	Palipase	ec
Liquibid 1200	sr	Palipase MT 16	ec
Liquibid-D	sr	Palipase MT 20	ec
Lithobid	sr	Palpeon DR 10	ec
Lodine XL	sr	Palpeon DR 20	ec
Lodrane 12 Hour	sr	Paltrase MT 20	ec
Lodrane LD	sr	Pancrease	ec
Mag Delay	sr	Pancrease MT 10	ec
Mag-SR	sr	Pancrease MT 16	ec
Mag-Tab SR	sr	Pancrease MT 20	ec
Maxifed	sr	Pancrecarb MS-4	ec
Maxifed DM	sr	Pancrecarb MS-8	ec
Maxifed-G	sr	Pancrelipase 16,000	ec
Maxovite	sr		
Medent DM	sr	Pancrelipase 20,000	ec
Medent LD	sr		
Med-Rx	sr	Pancron 10	ec
Med-Rx DM	sr	Pancron 20	ec
Mega-C	sr	Pangestyme CN-10	ec
Melfiat	sr		
Mescolor	sr	Pangestyme CN-20	ec
Mestinon Timespan		Pangestyme EC	ec
Metadate CD	sr	Pangestyme MT16	ec
Metadate ER	sr		
Methylin ER	sr	Pangestyme UL12	ec
Micro-K	sr		
Micro-K 10	sr	Pangestyme UL18	ec
Miraphen PSE	sr		
Modane	ec	Pangestyme UL20	ec
MS Contin	sr		
Muco-Fen	sr	Panmist DM	sr
Muco-Fen 1200	sr	Panmist JR	sr
Muco-Fen DM	sr	Panmist LA	sr
Multi-Ferrous Folic	sr	Pannaz	sr
		Papacon	sr
Multiret Folic-500	sr	Para-Time SR	sr
Nalex-A	sr	Paser	or
Naprelan	sr	Pavacot	sr
Nasabid SR	sr	PCE Dispertab	or
Nasatab LA	sr	Pentasa	sr
Nd Clear	sr	Pentopak	sr
Nexium	ec	Pentoxil	sr
Niacin Time-Release	sr	Pharmadrine	sr
		Phendiet-105	sr
Niaspan	sr	Plendil	sr
Nifedical XL	sr	Poly Hist Forte	sr
Nitrocot	sr	Poly-Vent	sr
Nitrogard	sr	Poly-Vent JR	sr
Nitroglyn E-R	sr	Prehist D	sr
Nitro-Time	sr	Prelu-2	sr
Norflex	sr		

(Continued on next page)

Drug	Type of Release	Drug	Manufacturer	Type of Release
Prevacid	ec	Rondec-TR		sr
Prilosec	ec	Sam-E		ec
Procanbid	sr	Sam-E		ec
Procardia XL	sr	Sinemet CR		sr
Profen Forte	sr	Sinuvent PE		sr
Profen Forte DM	sr	Slo-Niacin		sr
Profen II	sr	Slow Fe		sr
Profen II DM	sr	Slow Fe With Folic Acid		sr
Prohist-8	sr			
Prolex PD	sr	Slow-Mag		sr
Prolex-D	sr	Spacol T/S		sr
Pronestyl-SR	sr	S-Pak		sr
Propan	sr	S-Pak DM		sr
Protid	sr	St. Joseph Pain Reliever		ec
Protonix	ec			
Protuss-DM	sr	Stahist		sr
Proventil Repetabs	sr	Stamoist E		sr
Prozac Weekly	ec	Sudafed 12 Hour		sr
Pseubrom	sr	Sudal 60/500		sr
Pseubrom-PD	sr	Sudal DM		sr
Pseudochlor	sr	Sular		sr
Pseudocot-C	sr	Superoxide Dismutase (SOD)		ec
Pseudocot-G	sr			
Pseudo-G	sr	Sureprin 81		ec
Pseudo-G/PSI	sr	Symax-SR		sr
Pseudo-PD	sr	Tarka		sr
Pseudovent	sr	Tegretol-XR		sr
Pseudovent Ped	sr	Tenuate Dospan		sr
Q-Bid DM	sr	Theo-24		sr
Q-Bid LA	sr	Theochron		sr
Quadra-Hist D	sr	Theo-Time		sr
Quadra-Hist D Ped	sr	Thiamilate		ec
		Thorazine Spansule		sr
Quibron-T/SR	sr	Tiazac		sr
Quinaglute Dura-Tabs	sr	Time-Hist		sr
		Toprol XL		sr
Quindal	sr	Totalday		sr
Quinidex Extentabs	sr	Touro Allergy		sr
		Touro CC		sr
Regiprin	ec	Touro DM		sr
Reliable Gentle Laxative	ec	Touro EX		sr
		Touro LA		sr
Resbid	sr	T-Phyl		sr
Rescon	sr	Tranxene SD		sr
Rescon JR	sr	Trental		sr
Rescon MX	sr	Trinalin Repetabs		sr
Rescon-ED	sr	Tussafed-LA		sr
Respa-1st	sr	Tussi-Bid		sr
Respa-DM	sr	Tylenol Arthritis		sr
Respa-GF	sr	Ultrabrom		sr
Respahist	sr	Ultrabrom PD		sr
Respaire-120 SR	sr	Ultrase		ec
Respaire-60 SR	sr	Ultrase MT12		ec
Ribo-2	ec	Ultrase MT18		ec
Rinade-BID	sr	Ultrase MT20		ec
Ritalin-SR	sr	Uniphyl		sr
Rodex Forte	sr	Urimax		ec
Rondamine	sr	Urocit-K 10		sr

Drug	Type of Release	Drug	Type of Release
Urocit-K 5	sr	Voltaren	ec
Vanex Forte-D	sr	Voltaren-XR	sr
V-Dec-M	sr	We Mist LA	sr
Veracolate	ec	Wellbutrin SR	sr
Verelan	sr	Westrim LA	sr
Verelan PM	sr	Wobenzym N	ec
Versacaps	sr	Xiral	sr
Videx EC	ec	YSP Aspirin	ec
Vitamin C	sr	Zaptec PSE	sr
Timed-Release		Zephrex LA	sr
Vitamin C/Rose	sr	Zorprin	sr
Hips		Zyban	sr
Vitelle Irospan	sr	Zymase	ec
Vivotif Berna	ec	Zyrtec-D	sr
Volmax	sr		

[a]ec, enteric-coated; or, other; sr, slow-release.

Reprinted with permission from *The Drug Topics Red Book*. Thomson Medical Economics: Montvale, NJ, 2002.

Sugar-Free Products

Listed below, by therapeutic category, is a selection of drug products that contain no sugar. When recommending these products to diabetic patients, keep in mind that many may contain sorbitol, alcohol, or other sources of carbohydrates. This list should not be considered all-inclusive. Generics and alternate brands of some products may be available. Check product labeling for a current listing of inactive ingredients.

Product	Product

ANALGESICS
Actamin Maximum Strength Liquid
Aminofen Tablet
Aminofen Max Tablet
Aspirtab Tablet
Aspirtab Max Tablet
Back Pain-Off Tablet
Backprin Tablet
Buffasal Tablet
Buffasal Max Tablet
Dyspel Tablet
Febrol Liquid
Medi-Seltzer Effervescent Tablet
Ms.-Aid Tablet
Non-Aspirin Pain Relief Elixir
PMS Relief Tablet
Silapap Children's Elixir
Sureprin 81 Tablet

ANTACIDS/ANTIFLATULENTS
Almag Chewable Tablet
Alcalak Chewable Tablet
Aldroxicon I Suspension
Aldroxicon II Suspension
Baby Gasz Drops
Diabeti-Gest Tablet
Dimacid Chewable Tablet
Diotame Chewable Tablet
Diotame Liquid
Gas-Ban Chewable Tablet
Mallamint Chewable Tablet
Mylanta Gelcaplet
Neutralin Tablet
Pepto-Bismol Liquid
Pepto-Bismol Chewable Tablet
Riopan Plus Suspension
Riopan Suspension
Titralac Chewable Tablet
Titralac Plus Chewable Tablet
Tums E-X Chewable Tablet

(Continued on next page)

Product

ANTIASTHMATIC/RESPIRATORY AGENTS
Elixophyllin-GG Liquid
Jay-Phyl Syrup
Ventolin Syrup

ANTIDIARRHEALS
Diasorb Liquid
Diarrest Tablet
Di-Gon II Tablet
Donnagel Liquid
Imogen Liquid
Pepto-Bismol Liquid
Pepto-Bismol Chewable Tablet

BLOOD MODIFIERS/IRON PREPARATIONS
Diatx Fe Tablet
Iberet Liquid
I.L.X. B-12 Elixir
Irofol Liquid
Irofol Drops
Nephro-Fer Tablet
Niferex Elixir

CORTICOSTEROIDS
Prelone Syrup

COUGH/COLD/ALLERGY PREPARATIONS
Accuhist DM Pediatric Drops
Accuhist LA Tablet
Accuhist Pediatric Drops
Anaplex DM Syrup
Anaplex HD Syrup
Atuss EX Liquid
Biodec DM Drops
Biodec DM Syrup
Bromophed DX Syrup
B-Tuss Liquid
Carbofed DM Syrup
Carbofed DM Drops
Cepacol Sore Throat Children's Liquid
Cetafen Cold Tablet
Cheratussin DAC Liquid
Codal-DM Syrup
Codotuss Liquid
Coldonyl Tablet
Co-Tussin Liquid
Cotuss-V Syrup
Cytuss HC Syrup
D-Care Cough Syrup
Decorel Forte Tablet
Despec Liquid
Despec-SF Liquid
Diabetic Tussin Allergy Relief Liquid
Diabetic Tussin Allergy Relief Gelcaplet
Diabetic Tussin C Expectorant Liquid
Diabetic Tussin Children's Liquid
Diabetic Tussin Cold & Flu Gelcaplet
Diabetic Tussin DM Liquid
Diabetic Tussin DM Maximum Strength Liquid
Diabetic Tussin DM Maximum Strength Softgel

Product

Diabetic Tussin EX Liquid
Diabe-Tuss DM Liquid
Dimetapp Allergy Children's Elixir
Diphen Capsule
Double-Tussin DM Liquid
Duraganidin DM Liquid
Durahistine DM Syrup
Echotuss-HC Syrup
Endal Expectorant Liquid
Endal HD Liquid
Endal HD Plus Liquid
Endotuss-HD Syrup
Enplus-HD Syrup
Entex Syrup
Entex HC Syrup
Exo-Tuss Syrup
Gani-Tuss NR Liquid
Gani-Tuss-DM NR Liquid
Genecof-HC Liquid
Genecof-XP Liquid
Genedel Syrup
Genedotuss-DM Liquid
Genexpect DM Liquid
Genexpect-PE Liquid
Genexpect-SF Liquid
Giltuss Liquid
Giltuss HC Syrup
Giltuss Pediatric Liquid
Giltuss TR Tablet
Guai-Co Liquid
Guaicon DMS Liquid
Guai-DEX Liquid
Guiatuss AC Syrup
Guiatuss AC Syrup
Guiatuss DAC Syrup
Halotussin AC Liquid
Halotussin DAC Liquid
Hayfebrol Liquid
H-C Tussive Syrup
Histex PD Liquid
Histinex HC Syrup
Histinex PV Syrup
Hydro PC Syrup
Hydron KGS Liquid
Hydro-Tussin DM Elixir
Hydro-Tussin HC Syrup
Hydro-Tussin HD Liquid
Hyphen-HD Syrup
Hytuss Tablet
Hytuss 2X Capsule
Iofen-C NF Liquid
Iofen-DM NF Liquid
Iofen-NF Liquid
Iophen DM Liquid
Iotussin HC Liquid
Jaycof Expectorant Syrup
Jaycof-HC Liquid
Jaycof-XP Liquid
Kentuss Syrup

Product	Product
Kita LA Tos Liquid	Siladryl Allergy Liquid
Levall 5.0 Liquid	Siladryl DAS Liquid
Lodrane Liquid	Sildec Syrup
Marcof Expectorant Syrup	Sildec Drops
M-Clear Syrup	Sildec-DM Syrup
M-End Liquid	Sildec-DM Liquid
Mytussin AC Cough Syrup	Silexin Syrup
Mytussin DAC Syrup	Silexin Tablet
Nalex DH Liquid	Siltussin DAS Liquid
Nalex-A Liquid	Siltussin DM DAS Cough Formula Syrup
Nalspan Senior DX Liquid	Siltussin SA Syrup
Neotuss S/F Liquid	S-T Forte 2 Liquid
Neotuss-D liquid	Super Tussin DM Liquid
Norel DM Liquid	Supress DX Pediatric Drops
Nycoff Tablet	Suttar-SF Syrup
Onset Forte Tablet	Tricodene Syrup
Orgadin Liquid	Trispec-PE Liquid
Orgadin-Tuss Liquid	Tussafed Syrup
Orgadin-Tuss DM Liquid	Tussafed-EX Pediatric Drops
Organidin NR Liquid	Tussafed-HC Syrup
Organidin NR Tablet	Tussaphen DM Syrup
Palgic-DS Syrup	Tuss-DM Liquid
Pancof HC Liquid	Tuss-ES Syrup
Pancof XP Liquid	Tussi-Organidin DM NR Liquid
Panmist DM Syrup	Tussi-Organidin DM-S NR Liquid
Pediatex Liquid	Tussi-Organidin NR Liquid
Pediatex DM Liquid	Tussi-Organidin-S NR Liquid
Pediatex-D Liquid	Tussi-Pres Liquid
Phanasin Syrup	Tussirex Liquid
Phanasin Diabetic Choice Syrup	Vicks Dayquil Multi- Symptom Liquicap
Phanatuss Syrup	Vicodin Tuss Expectorant Syrup
Pneumotussin 2.5 Syrup	Vi-Q-Tuss Syrup
Poly-Tussin Syrup	Vitussin Expectorant Syrup
Poly-Tussin DM Syrup	Vortex Syrup
Poly-Tussin HD Syrup	Z-Cof DM Syrup
Poly-Tussin XP Syrup	Zyrtec Syrup
Pro-Cof Liquid	
Pro-Cof D Liquid	**FLUORIDE PREPARATIONS**
Profen II DM Solution	D-Care Baking Soda Toothpaste
Prolex DH Liquid	D-Care Tartar Control Toothpaste
Prolex DM Liquid	Fluorabon Tablet
Protuss Liquid	Fluor-A-Day Tablet
Protuss-D Liquid	Fluor-A-Day Lozenge
Robafen DAC Syrup	Flura-Loz Tablet
Robitussin-DAC Syrup	Lozi-Flur Lozenge
Romilar AC Liquid	Sensodyne w/Fluoride Gel
Romilar DM Liquid	Sensodyne w/Fluoride Tartar Control Toothpaste
Rondec Syrup	Sensodyne w/Fluoride Toothpaste
Rondec DM Syrup	
Rondec DM Drops	**LAXATIVES**
Ru Tuss-DM Syrup	Citrucel Powder
Scot-Tussin Allergy Relief Formula Liquid	Fiber Ease Liquid
Scot-Tussin DM Liquid	Fibro-XL Capsule
Scot-Tussin DM Cough Chasers Lozenge	Konsyl Easy Mix Formula Powder
Scot-Tussin Expectorant Liquid	Konsyl-Orange Powder
Scot-Tussin Original Liquid	Metamucil Smooth Texture Powder
Scot-Tussin Senior Liquid	Reguloid Powder

(Continued on next page)

Product

MISCELLANEOUS
Acidoll Capsule
Alka-Gest Tablet
Bicitra Solution
Colidrops Pediatric Drops
Cytra-2 Solution
Cytra-K Solution
Cytra-K Crystals
Melatin Tablet
Neutra-Phos Powder
Neutra-Phos-K Powder
Polycitra-K Solution
Polycitra-LC Solution
Questran Light Powder
Rhogam Solution

MOUTH/THROAT PREPARATIONS
Benloz Extra Strength Lozenges
Cepacol Maximum Strength Spray
Cepacol Sore Throat Lozenges
Cheracol Sore Throat Spray
Cylex Lozenges
Diabetic Tussin Cough Drops
Diabetirinse Solution
Fisherman's Friend Lozenges
Fresh N Free Liquid
Isodettes Sore Throat Spray
Larynex Lozenges
Medikoff Drops
N'Ice Lozenges
Ocusurg Powder
Oragesic Solution
Orasept Mouthwash/ Gargle Liquid
Robitussin Lozenges
Sepasoothe Lozenges
Spritz Mouthwash Powder
Thorets Maximum Strength Lozenges
Throtoceptic Spray
Vademecum Mouthwash & Gargle Concentrate

POTASSIUM SUPPLEMENTS
Cena K Liquid
Kaon Elixir
Kaon-Cl 20% Liquid
Kay Ciel Powder
Klor-Con/25 Powder
Klor-Con/EF Tablet
Rum-K Liquid

VITAMINS/MINERALS/SUPPLEMENTS
Action-Tabs Made For Men
Adaptosode For Stress Liquid
Adaptosode R+R For Acute Stress Liquid
Amino Acid Complex Tablet
Aminoplex Powder
Aminostasis Powder
Aminotate Powder
B-C-Bid Caplet
Bevitamel Tablet
Biosode Liquid

Product

Biotect Plus Caplet
Bugs Bunny Complete Chewable Tablet
Bugs Bunny w/Extra Vitamin C Chewable Tablet
Bugs Bunny w/Iron Chewable Tablet
C & M Caps-375 Capsule
Calbon Tablet
Cal-Cee Tablet
Cal-Mint Chewable Tablet
Carox Plus Tablet
Cevi-Bid Tablet
Cholestratin Tablet
Chromacaps Tablet
Chromium K6 Tablet
Combi-Cart Tablet
Complete 2000 Capsule
Daily Herbs Formulas
D-Care Meal
    Replacement
D-Care Snack
Delta D3 Tablet
Detoxosode Liquid
DHEA Capsule
Diatx Tablet
Diet System 6 Gum
Diucaps Capsule
DI-Phen-500 Capsule
Electrotab Tablet
Endorphenyl Capsule
Enfagrow Oatmeal
Enterex Diabetic Liquid
Essential Nutrients Plus Silica Tablet
Evolve Softgel
Ex-L Tablet
Extress Tablet
Eyetamins Tablet
Fem Cal Tablet
Folacin-800 Tablet
Foltx Tablet
Gram-O-Leci Tablet
Hemovit Tablet
Herbal Slim Complex Capsule
Legatrin GCM Formula Tablet
Lynae Calcium/Vitamin C Chewable Tablet
Lynae Chondroitin/ Glucosamine Capsule
Lynae Ginse-Cool Chewable Tablet
Mag-Caps Capsule
Mag-Ox 400 Tablet
Mag-SR Tablet
New Life Hair Tablet
Nutrisure OTC Tablet
O-Cal Fa Tablet
Plenamins Plus Tablet
Powermate Tablet
Prostaplex Herbal Complex Capsule
Prostatonin Capsule
Protect Plus Liquid
Protect Plus Softgel
Quintabs-M Tablet
Re/Neph Liquid
Releaf For PMS Tablet

Product

Replace Capsule
Replace w/o Iron Capsule
Resource Arginaid Powder
Ribo-100 T.D. Capsule
Samolinic Softgel
Sea Omega 30 Softgel
Sea Omega 50 Softgel
Strovite Forte Syrup
Sunnie Tablet
Sunvite Tablet
Sunvite Platinum Tablet
Suplevit Liquid
Theraplex Liquid

Product

Triamin Tablet
Triamino Tablet
Tums Calcium For Life PMS Tablet
Ultramino Powder
Uro-Mag Capsule
Vitalize Liquid
Vitamin C/Rose Hips Tablet
Vitrum Jr Chewable Tablet
Xtramins Tablet
Yohimbe Power Max 1500 For Women Tablet
Yohimbized 1000 Capsule
Ze-Plus Softgel

Reprinted with permission from *The Drug Topics Red Book*. Thomson Medical Economics: Montvale, NJ, 2002.

Alcohol-Free Products

The following is a selection of alcohol-free products grouped by therapeutic category. The list is not comprehensive. Generic and alternate brands may exist. Always check product labeling for definitive information on specific ingredients.

Product

ANALGESICS
Acetaminophen Infants Drops
Actamin Maximum Strength Liquid
Advil Children's Suspension
Aminofen Tablet
Aminofen Max Tablet
APAP Elixir
Aspirtab Tablet
Aspirtab Max Tablet
Buffasal Tablet
Buffasal Max Tablet
Demerol Hydrochloride Syrup
Dolono Elixir
Dolono Infants Drops
Dyspel Tablet
Genapap Children Elixir
Genapap Infant's Drops
Motrin Children's Suspension
Silapap Children's Elixir
Silapap Infant's Drops
Tempra 1 Drops
Tempra 2 Syrup
Tylenol Children's Suspension
Tylenol Infant's Drops

ANTIASTHMATIC AGENTS
Dilor-G Liquid
Dy-G Liquid
Elixophyllin-GG Liquid

ANTICONVULSANTS
Zarontin Syrup

ANTIVIRAL AGENTS
Epivir Oral Solution

Product

COUGH/COLD/ALLERGY PREPARATIONS
Accuhist Pediatric Drops
Allergy Relief Medicine Children's Elixir
Anaplex DM Syrup
Anaplex HD Syrup
Andehist DM Drops
Andehist DM Syrup
Atuss DM Liquid
Atuss EX Liquid
Atuss G Liquid
Atuss MS Syrup
Biodec DM Drops
Biodec DM Syrup
Bromaline Solution
Bromaline DM Elixir
Bromanate Elixir
Bron-Tuss Liquid
B-Tuss Liquid
Carbatuss Liquid
Carbofed DM Drops
Carbofed DM Syrup
Cepacol Sore Throat Children's Liquid
Chlor-Trimeton Allergy Syrup
Codal-DH Syrup
Codal-DM Syrup
Codotuss Liquid
Coldonyl Tablet
Complete Allergy Elixir
Co-Tussin Liquid
Cotuss-V Syrup
Creomulsion Complete Syrup
Creomulsion Cough Syrup
Creomulsion For Children Syrup
Creomulsion Pediatric Syrup

(Continued on next page)

Product

Cytuss HC Syrup
D-Care Cough Syrup
Dehistine Syrup
Deltuss Liquid
Despec Liquid Labs
Diabetic Tussin Allergy Relief Liquid
Diabetic Tussin Allergy Relief Tablet
Diabetic Tussin C Expectorant Liquid
Diabetic Tussin Children's Liquid
Diabetic Tussin Cold & Flu Tablet
Diabetic Tussin DM Liquid
Diabetic Tussin DM Maximum Strength Liquid
Diabetic Tussin DM Maximum Strength Capsule
Diabetic Tussin EX Liquid
Diabe-Tuss DM Syrup
Dimetapp Allergy Children's Elixir
Dimetapp Cold & Fever Children's Suspension
Dimetapp Decongestant Pediatric Drops
Double-Tussin DM Liquid
Duraganidin DM Liquid
Durahistine DM Syrup
Echotuss-HC Syrup
Endagen-HD Syrup
Endal HD Syrup
Endal HD Plus Syrup
Endotuss-HD Syrup
Enplus-HD Syrup
Entex Syrup
Entex HC Syrup
Exo-Tuss
Father John's Medicine Plus Drops
Friallergia DM Liquid
Friallergia Liquid
Gani-Tuss NR Liquid
Gani-Tuss-DM NR Liquid
Genahist Elixir
Giltuss HC Syrup
Giltuss Liquid
Giltuss Pediatric Liquid
Guai-Co Liquid
Guaicon DMS Liquid
Guai-Dex Liquid
Guaifed Syrup
Guiatuss CF Syrup
Halotussin Syrup
Hayfebrol Liquid
H-C Tussive Syrup
Histex Liquid
Histex PD Drops
Histex PD Liquid
Histinex HC Syrup
Histinex PV Syrup
Hycomal DH Liquid
Hydone Liquid
Hydramine Elixir
Hydro-Tussin DM Elixir
Hydro-Tussin HC Syrup
Hydro-Tussin HD Liquid
Hyphen-HD Syrup
Iodal HD Liquid

Product

Iofen-C NF Liquid
Iofen-DM NF Liquid
Iofen-NF Liquid
Iophen DM Liquid
Iotussin HC Liquid
Jaycof Expectorant Syrup
Jaycof-HC Liquid
Jaycof-XP Liquid
Kentuss Syrup
KG-Dal HD Plus Syrup
Kita La Tos Liquid
Levall Liquid
Levall 5.0 Liquid
Lodrane Liquid
Marcof Expectorant Syrup
M-Clear Syrup
Medi-Brom Elixir
M-End Liquid
Motrin Cold Children's Suspension
Mytussin-PE Liquid
Nalex DH Liquid
Nalex-A Liquid
Nalspan Senior DX Liquid
Neotuss S/F Liquid
Neotuss-D Liquid
Norel DM Liquid
Nucofed Syrup
Nycoff Tablet
Orgadin Liquid
Orgadin-Tuss Liquid
Orgadin-Tuss DM Liquid
Organidin NR Liquid
Palgic-DS Syrup
Pancof HC Liquid
Pancof XP Liquid
Panmist DM Syrup
Panmist-S Syrup
Pediacare Cold + Allergy Children's Liquid
Pediacare Cough-Cold Liquid
Pediacare Decongestant Infants Drops
Pediacare Decongestant Plus Cough Drops
Pediacare Multi-Symptom Liquid
Pediacare Nightrest Liquid
Pedia-Relief Liquid
Pediatex Liquid
Pediatex-D Liquid
Phanasin Syrup
Phanatuss Syrup
Pharmasin Syrup
Pharmatuss DM Syrup
Phena-S Liquid
Pneumotussin 2.5 Syrup
Poly-Tussin Syrup
Poly-Tussin DM Syrup
Poly-Tussin HD Syrup
Poly-Tussin XP Syrup
Primsol Solution
Pro-Cof Liquid
Profen II DM Liquid
Prolex DH Liquid

Product

Prolex DM Liquid
Protuss Liquid
Protuss-D Liquid
Q-Tussin PE Liquid
Robitussin Cough & Congestion Liquid
Robitussin DM Syrup
Robitussin PE Syrup
Robitussin Pediatric Drops
Robitussin Pediatric Cough Syrup
Robitussin Pediatric Night Relief Liquid
Romilar AC Liquid
Romilar DM Liquid
Rondec Syrup
Rondec DM Drops
Rondec DM Syrup
Scot-Tussin Allergy Relief Formula Liquid
Scot-Tussin DM Liquid
Scot-Tussin Expectorant Liquid
Scot-Tussin Original Syrup
Scot-Tussin Senior Liquid
Siladryl Allergy Liquid
Siladryl DAS Liquid
Sildec Liquid
Sildec Syrup
Sildec-DM Drops
Sildec-DM Syrup
Siltussin DAS Liquid
Siltussin DM Syrup
Siltussin DM DAS Cough Formula Syrup
Siltussin SA Syrup
S-T Forte 2 Liquid
Sudatuss DM Syrup
Sudatuss-2 Liquid
Sudatuss-SF Liquid
Super Tussin DM Liquid
Triaminic Infant Decongestant Drops
Trispec-PE Liquid
Tussafed Syrup
Tussafed-EX Syrup
Tussafed-EX Pediatric Liquid
Tussafed-HC Syrup
Tuss-DM Liquid
Tuss-ES Syrup
Tussi-Organidin DM NR Liquid
Tussi-Organidin DM-S NR Liquid
Tussi-Organidin NR Liquid
Tussi-Organidin-S NR Liquid
Tussi-Pres Liquid
Tussirex Liquid
Tussirex Syrup
Tylenol Allergy-D Children's Liquid
Tylenol Cold Children's Liquid
Tylenol Cold Infants Drops
Tylenol Cold Plus Cough Children's Liquid
Tylenol Flu Children's Suspension
Tylenol Flu Night Time Max Strength Liquid
Tylenol Sinus Children's Liquid
Vanex-HD Syrup
Vicks 44E Pediatric Liquid
Vicks 44M Pediatric Liquid

Product

Vicks Dayquil Multi-Symptom Liquicap
Vicks Dayquil Multi-Symptom Liquid
Vicks Nyquil Children's Liquid
Vicodin Tuss Expectorant Syrup
Vi-Q-Tuss Syrup
Vitussin Expectorant Syrup
Vortex Syrup
Z-Cof DM Syrup

EAR/NOSE/THROAT PRODUCTS
4-Way Saline Moisturizing Mist Spray
Ayr Baby Saline Spray
Bucalsep Solution
Bucalsep Spray
Cheracol Sore Throat Spray
Diabetirinse Solution
Fresh N Free Liquid
Glandosane Solution
Gly-Oxide Liquid
Isodettes Sore Throat Spray
Lacrosse Mouthwash Liquid
Larynex Lozenges
Listermint Liquid
Nasal Moist Gel
Orajel Baby Liquid
Orajel Baby Nighttime Gel
Orasept Mouthwash/ Gargle Liquid
Spritz Mouthwash Powder
Tanac Liquid
Tech 2000 Dental Rinse Liquid
Throto-Ceptic Spray
Zilactin Baby Extra Strength Gel

GASTROINTESTINAL AGENTS
Agoral Liquid
Baby Gasz Drops
Colace Liquid
Colidrops Pediatric Drops
Diarrest Tablet
Imogen Liquid
Kaodene NN Suspension
Kaopectate Advanced Formula Suspension
Kaopectate Children's Liquid Suspension
Liqui-Doss Liquid
Mylicon Infants' Suspension
Neoloid Liquid
Neutralin Tablet
Senokot Children's Syrup

HEMATINICS
Feostat Suspension
Irofol Liquid

MISCELLANEOUS
Cytra-2 Solution
Cytra-K Solution
Emetrol Solution
Emetrol Solution
Fluorinse Solution
Rum-K Liquid

(Continued on next page)

Product	Product
PSYCHOTROPICS	**VITAMINS/MINERALS/SUPPLEMENTS**
Thorazine Syrup	Adaptosode For Stress Liquid
	Adaptosode R+R For Acute Stress Liquid
TOPICAL PRODUCTS	Biosode Liquid
Aloe Vesta 2-N-1 Antifungal Ointment	Detoxosode Products Liquid
Fleet Pain Relief Pads	Genesupp-500 Liquid
Fresh & Pure Douche Solution	Genetect Plus Liquid
Handclens Solution	Multi-Delyn w/Iron Liquid
Klenz Kloth Pads	Poly-Vi-Sol Drops
Lid Wipes-SPF Pads	Poly-Vi-Sol w/Iron Drops
Neutrogena Acne Wash Liquid	Protect Plus Liquid
Neutrogena Antiseptic Liquid	Soluvite-F Drops
Neutrogena Clear Pore Gel	Strovite Forte Syrup
Neutrogena T/Derm Liquid	Suplevit Liquid
Neutrogena Toner Liquid	Theragran Liquid
Podiclens Spray	Theraplex Liquid
Propa PH Foaming Face Wash Liquid	Tri-Vi-Sol Drops
Sea Breeze Foaming Face Wash Gel	Tri-Vi-Sol w/Iron Drops
Stri-Dex Pad	Vitafol Syrup
Stri-Dex Maximum Strength Pad	Vitalize Liquid
Stri-Dex Sensitive Skin Pad	Vitamin C/Rose Hips Tablet, Extended Release
Stri-Dex Super Scrub Pad	

Reprinted with permission from *The Drug Topics Red Book*. Thomson Medical Economics: Montvale, NJ, 2002.

Drugs That May Cause Photosensitivity

The drugs in this table are known to cause photosensitivity in some individuals. Effects can range from itching, scaling, rash, and swelling to skin cancer, premature skin aging, skin and eye burns, cataracts, reduced immunity, blood vessel damage, and allergic reactions. The list is not all-inclusive, and shows only representative brands of each generic. When in doubt, always check specific product labeling. Individuals should be advised to wear protective clothing and to apply sunscreens while taking the medications listed below.

Generic	Brand	Generic	Brand
Acetazolamide	Diamox	Bendroflumethiazide/ nadolol	Corzide
Acitretin	Soriatane		
Alendronate	Fosamax	Bexarotene	Targretin
Alitretinoin	Panretin	Bismuth/metronidazole/ tetracycline	Helidac
Amiloride/ hydrochlorothiazide	Moduretic		
		Bisoprolol/ hydrochlorothiazide	Ziac
Amiodarone	Cordarone, Pacerone	Brompheniramine/ dextromethorphan/ pseudoephedrine	Bromfed-DM, Dimetane-DX
Amitriptyline	Elavil		
Amitriptyline/ chlordiazepoxide	Limbitrol	Bupropion	Wellbutrin, Zyban
		Candesartan/ hydrochlorothiazide	Atacand HCT
Amitriptyline/perphenazine	Etrafon, Etrafon-Forte, Triavil		
		Capecitabine	Xeloda
Amoxapine		Captopril	Capoten
Anagrelide	Agrylin	Captopril/ hydrochlorothiazide	Capozide
Atenolol/chlorthalidone	Tenoretic		
Atorvastatin	Lipitor	Carbamazepine	Carbatrol, Tegretol, Tegretol-XR
Aurothioglucose	Solganal		
Azatadine/pseudoephedrine	Rynatan, Trinalin	Carbinoxamine/ pseudoephedrine	Palgic-D, Palgic-DS, Pediatex-D
Azithromycin	Zithromax		
Benazepril	Lotensin	Carvedilol	Coreg
Benazepril/ hydrochlorothiazide	Lotensin HCT	Celecoxib	Celebrex

Generic	Brand	Generic	Brand
Cetirizine	Zyrtec	Fluvastatin	Lescol
Cevimeline	Evoxac	Fluvoxamine	Luvox
Chlorhexidine gluconate	Hibistat	Fosinopril	Monopril
Chlorothiazide	Diuril	Fosphenytoin	Cerebyx
Chlorpheniramine/ hydrocodone/ pseudoephedrine	Tussend	Furosemide	Lasix
		Gabapentin	Neurontin
		Gatifloxacin	Tequin
Chlorpheniramine/ phenylephrine/pyrilamine	Rynatan	Gemfibrozil	Lopid
		Gentamicin	Garamycin
Chlorpromazine	Thorazine	Glatiramer	Copaxone
Chlorpropamide	Diabinese	Glimepiride	Amaryl
Chlorthalidone	Thalitone	Glipizide	Glucotrol
Chlorthalidone/clonidine	Combipres	Glyburide	DiaBeta, Glynase, Micronase
Cidofovir	Vistide		
Ciprofloxacin	Cipro	Glyburide/metformin HCl	Glucovance
Citalopram	Celexa	Griseofulvin	Fulvicin P/G, Grifulvin, Gris-PEG
Clemastine	Tavist		
Clozapine	Clozaril		
Cromolyn sodium	Gastrocrom	Haloperidol	Haldol
Cyclobenzaprine	Flexeril	Hexachlorophene	pHisoHex
Cyproheptadine	Periactin	Hydralazine/ hydrochlorothiazide	Apresazide
Dacarbazine	DTIC-Dome		
Dantrolene	Dantrium	Hydrochlorothiazide	HydroDIURIL, Hyzaar, Microzide, Oretic
Demeclocycline	Declomycin		
Desipramine	Norpramin		
Diclofenac potassium	Cataflam		
Diclofenac sodium	Voltaren, Voltaren-XR	Hydrochlorothiazide/ fosinopril	Monopril HCT
Diclofenac sodium/ misoprostol	Arthrotec	Hydrochlorothiazide/ irbesartan	Avalide
Diflunisal	Dolobid	Hydrochlorothiazide/ lisinopril	Prinzide, Zestoretic
Dihydroergotamine	D.H.E. 45		
Diltiazem	Cardizem, Tiazac	Hydrochlorothiazide/ losartan potassium	Hyzaar
Diphenhydramine	Benadryl		
Divalproex	Depakote	Hydrochlorothiazide/ methyldopa	Aldoril
Doxepin	Sinequan		
Doxycycline hyclate	Doryx, Periostat, Vibra-Tabs, Vibramycin	Hydrochlorothiazide/ moexipril	Uniretic
		Hydrochlorothiazide/ propranolol	Inderide
Doxycycline monohydrate	Monodox		
Enalapril	Vasotec	Hydrochlorothiazide/ quinapril	Accuretic
Enalapril/felodipine	Lexxel		
Enalapril/ hydrochlorothiazide	Vaseretic	Hydrochlorothiazide/ spironolactone	Aldactazide
Enalaprilat	Vasotec I.V.	Hydrochlorothiazide/ telmisartan	Micardis HCT
Enoxacin	Penetrex		
Epirubicin	Ellence	Hydrochlorothiazide/ timolol	Timolide
Erythromycin/sulfisoxazole	Pediazole		
Estazolam	ProSom	Hydrochlorothiazide/ triamterene	Dyazide, Maxzide
Estradiol	Gynodiol		
Ethionamide	Trecator-SC	Hydrochlorothiazide/ valsartan	Diovan HCT
Etodolac	Lodine		
Felbamate	Felbatol	Hydroflumethiazide	Diucardin
Fenofibrate	Tricor	Hypericum	Kira, St. John's Wort
Floxuridine	Sterile FUDR		
Flucytosine	Ancobon	Hypericum/vitamin B_1/ vitamin C/kava-kava	One-A-Day Tension & Mood
Fluorouracil	Efudex		
Fluoxetine	Prozac, Sarafem	Ibuprofen	Motrin
Fluphenazine	Prolixin	Imipramine	Tofranil
Flutamide	Eulexin		

(Continued on next page)

Generic	Brand	Generic	Brand
Indapamide	Lozol	Pimpinella major	Burnet
Interferon alfa-2b, recombinant	Intron A	Piroxicam	Feldene
		Polymyxin B/trimethoprim	Polytrim
Interferon alfa-n3 (human leukocyte derived)	Alferon-N	Polythiazide	Renese
		Polythiazide/prazosin	Minizide
Interferon beta-1a	Avonex	Porfimer sodium	Photofrin
Interferon beta-1b	Betaseron	Pravastatin	Pravachol
Irbesartan/ hydrochlorothiazide	Avalide	Prochlorperazine	Compazine, Compro
Isoniazid/pyrazinamide/ rifampin	Rifater	Promethazine	Phenergan
		Protriptyline	Vivactil
Ketoprofen	Orudis, Oruvail	Pyrazinamide	Pyrazinamide
Lamotrigine	Lamictal	Quetiapine	Seroquel
Leuprolide	Lupron	Quinapril	Accupril
Levamisole	Ergamisol	Quinidine gluconate	Quinaglute, Quinidine
Lisinopril	Prinivil, Zestril		
Lomefloxacin	Maxaquin	Quinidine sulfate	Quinidex
Loratadine	Claritin	Rabeprazole sodium	Aciphex
Loratadine/ pseudoephedrine	Claritin-D	Ramipril	Altace
		Riluzole	Rilutek
Losartan	Cozaar	Risperidone	Risperdal
Lovastatin	Mevacor	Ritonavir	Norvir
Maprotiline	Ludiomil	Rizatriptan	Maxalt, Maxalt-MLT
Mefenamic acid	Ponstel		
Meloxicam	Mobic	Ropinirole	Requip
Meperidine/promethazine	Mepergan	Ruta graveolens	Rue
Mesalamine	Pentasa	Saquinavir	Fortovase
Methazolamide	Neptazane	Saquinavir mesylate	Invirase
Methotrexate	Trexall	Selegiline	Eldepryl
Methoxsalen	Uvadex, Oxsoralen	Sertraline	Zoloft
Methyclothiazide	Enduron	Sibutramine	Meridia
Metolazone	Mykrox, Zaroxolyn	Sildenafil	Viagra
Minocycline	Dynacin, Minocin	Simvastatin	Zocor
Mirtazapine	Remeron	Somatropin	Serostim
Moexipril	Univasc	Sotalol	Betapace, Betapace AF
Moxifloxacin	Avelox		
Nabumetone	Relafen	Sparfloxacin	Zagam
Nalidixic acid	NegGram	Sulfamethoxazole/ trimethoprim	Bactrim, Septra
Naproxen	Naprosyn, EC-Naprosyn	Sulfasalazine	Azulfidine
		Sulfisoxazole	Gantrisin Pediatric
Naproxen sodium	Anaprox, Naprelan	Sulindac	Clinoril
Naratriptan	Amerge	Sumatriptan	Imitrex
Nefazodone	Serzone	Tacrolimus	Prograf, Protopic
Nifedipine	Procardia	Tazarotene	Tazorac
Nisoldipine	Sular	Tetracycline	Achromycin
Norfloxacin	Noroxin	Thalidomide	Thalomid
Nortriptyline	Pamelor	Thioridazine hydrochloride	Mellaril
Ofloxacin	Floxin	Thiothixene	Navane
Olanzapine	Zyprexa, Zyprexa Zydis	Tiagabine	Gabitril
		Topiramate	Topamax
Olsalazine	Dipentum	Triamcinolone	Azmacort
Oxaprozin	Daypro	Triamterene	Dyrenium
Oxcarbazepine	Trileptal	Trifluoperazine	Stelazine
Oxytetracycline	Terramycin	Trimipramine	Surmontil
Paroxetine	Paxil	Trovafloxacin	Trovan
Pastinaca sativa	Parsnip	Valacyclovir	Valtrex
Pentosan polysulfate	Elmiron	Valproate	Depacon
Pentostatin	Nipent	Valproic acid	Depakene
Perphenazine	Trilafon	Venlafaxine	Effexor
Pilocarpine	Salagen		

Generic	Brand	Generic	Brand
Verteporfin	Visudyne	Ziprasidone	Geodon
Vinblastine		Zolmitriptan	Zomig
Zalcitabine	Hivid	Zolpidem	Ambien
Zaleplon	Sonata		

Reprinted with permission from *The Drug Topics Red Book*. Thomson Medical Economics: Montvale, NJ, 2002.

Drug–Alcohol Interactions

The following information was extracted from PharmaCIS™, the new *Clinical Integration System for Drug Utilization Review*™ from Red Book Database Services. The PharmaCIS database modules cover the full range of Omnibus Reconciliation Act requirements for drug utilization review, including the production of leaflets for patient education and screening for drug–drug interactions, previous allergies, therapeutic duplication, and improper dosing.

For further information on integrating PharmaCIS into an existing pharmacy system, contact your system vendor or Red Book Database Services at 800-722-3062.

Products are listed alphabetically, with summary warning statements given for each interaction. Degrees of onset and severity are indicated as follows. Onset: 1 = rapid (within 24 hours); 2 = delayed (after 24 hours). Severity: 1 = major (possibly life-threatening or potential permanent damage); 2 = moderate (may exacerbate the patient's condition); 3 = minor (little, if any, clinical effect).

Product	Interaction	Onset	Severity
Acetaminophen	Concurrent use of Ethanol and Acetaminophen may result in an increased risk of hepatotoxicity.	2	2
Acetophenazine	Concurrent use of Acetophenazine and Ethanol may result in increased central nervous system depression and an increased risk of extrapyramidal reactions.	1	2
Acitretin	Concurrent use of Acitretin and Ethanol may result in a prolonged risk of teratogenicity.	2	1
Alfentanil	Concurrent use of Ethanol and Alfentanil may result in decreased therapeutic effects for alfentanil.	2	2
Alprazolam	Concurrent use of Ethanol and Alprazolam may result in increased sedation.	1	2
Amitriptyline	Concurrent use of Ethanol and Amitriptyline may result in enhanced CNS depression and impairment of motor skills.	1	2
Amobarbital	Concurrent use of Ethanol and Amobarbital may result in excessive CNS depression.	1	2
Amoxapine	Concurrent use of Ethanol and Amoxapine may result in Ethanol enhanced drowsiness; impairment of motor skills.	1	2
Amprenavir	Concurrent use of Amprenavir and Ethanol may result in an increased risk of propylene glycol toxicity (seizures, tachycardia, lactic acidosis, renal toxicity, hemolysis).	2	1
Aprobarbital	Concurrent use of Aprobarbital and Ethanol may result in excessive CNS depression.	1	2
Aspirin	Concurrent use of Ethanol and Aspirin may result in increased gastrointestinal blood loss.	1	2
Bupropion	Concurrent use of Bupropion and Ethanol may result in an Ethanol increased risk of seizures.	2	1
Butabarbital	Concurrent use of Butabarbital and Ethanol may result in excessive CNS depression.	1	2
Butalbital	Concurrent use of Butalbital and Ethanol may result in excessive CNS depression.	1	2
Cefamandole	Concurrent use of Ethanol and Cefamandole may result in disulfiram-like reactions.	2	1
Cefmenoxime	Concurrent use of Ethanol and Cefmenoxime may result in disulfiram-like reactions.	1	1

(Continued on next page)

Product	Interaction	Onset	Severity
Cefoperazone	Concurrent use of Ethanol and Cefoperazone may result in l disulfiram-like reactions.	2	1
Cefotetan	Concurrent use of Ethanol and Cefotetan may result in disulfiram-like reactions.	2	1
Chloral hydrate	Concurrent use of Ethanol and Chloral Hydrate may result in increased sedation.	1	3
Chloral hydrate	Concurrent use of Ethanol and Chlordiazepoxide may result in increased sedation.	1	2
Chlorpromazine	Concurrent use of Ethanol and Chlorpromazine may result in increased sedation.	1	2
Chlorpropamide	Concurrent use of Ethanol and Chlorpropamide may result in disulfiram-like reactions.	1	1
Cimetidine	Concurrent use of Ethanol and Cimetidine may result in increased ethanol concentrations.	1	3
Cisapride	Concurrent use of Cisapride and Ethanol may result in increased blood levels of ethanol.	1	2
Clomipramine	Concurrent use of Ethanol and Clomipramine may result in enhanced drowsiness; impairment of motor skills.	1	2
Clorazepate	Concurrent use of Ethanol and Clorazepate may result in increased sedation.	1	2
Cocaine	Concurrent use of Ethanol and Cocaine may result in increased heart rate and blood pressure.	1	2
Codeine	Concurrent use of Ethanol and Codeine may result in increased sedation.	1	2
Cycloserine	Concurrent use of Cycloserine and Ethanol may result in an increased risk of seizures.	1	1
Desipramine	Concurrent use of Ethanol and Desipramine may result in enhanced drowsiness; impairment of motor skills.	1	2
Diazepam	Concurrent use of Ethanol and Diazepam may result in increased sedation.	1	2
Dimethindene	Concurrent use of Dimethindene and Ethanol may result in increased sedation.	1	2
Diphenhydramine	Concurrent use of Ethanol and Diphenhydramine may result in increased sedation.	1	2
Disulfiram	Concurrent use of Ethanol and Disulfiram may result in ethanol intolerance.	1	1
Dothiepin	Concurrent use of Ethanol and Dothiepin may result in enhanced drowsiness; impairment of motor skills.	1	2
Doxepin	Concurrent use of Ethanol and Doxepin may result in enhanced drowsiness; impairment of motor skills.	1	2
Eterobarb	Concurrent use of Eterobarb and Ethanol may result in excessive CNS depression.	1	2
Ethopropazine	Concurrent use of Ethopropazine and Ethanol may result in increased central nervous system depression and an increased risk of extrapyramidal reactions.	1	2
Flunitrazepam	Concurrent use of Flunitrazepam and Ethanol may result in excessive sedation and psychomotor impairment.	1	2
Fluphenazine	Concurrent use of Fluphenazine and Ethanol may result in increased central nervous system depression and an increased risk of extrapyramidal reactions.	1	2
Fomepizole	Concurrent use of Fomepizole and Ethanol may result in the reduced elimination of both drugs.	2	2
Fosphenytoin	Concurrent use of Fosphenytoin and Ethanol may result in decreased phenytoin serum concentrations, increased seizure potential, and additive CNS depressant effects.	1	2
Furazolidone	Concurrent use of Ethanol and Furazolidone may result in disulfiram-like reactions.	1	1
Gliclazide	Concurrent use of Ethanol and Gliclazide may result in prolonged hypoglycemia, disulfiram-like reactions.	1	1

Product	Interaction	Onset	Severity
Glipizide	Concurrent use of Ethanol and Glipizide may result in prolonged hypoglycemia, disulfiram-like reactions.	1	1
Glutethimide	Concurrent use of Ethanol and Glutethimide may result in increased sedation.	1	2
Glyburide	Concurrent use of Ethanol and Glyburide may result in prolonged hypoglycemia, disulfiram-like reactions.	1	1
Griseofulvin	Concurrent use of Griseofulvin and Ethanol may result in disulfiram-like reactions (nausea, vomiting, diarrhea, flushing, tachycardia, hypotension).	1	1
Hydrocodone	Concurrent use of Ethanol and Hydrocodone may result in increased sedation.	1	2
Hydromorphone	Concurrent use of Hydromorphone and Ethanol may result in increased sedation.	1	2
Imipramine	Concurrent use of Ethanol and Imipramine may result in enhanced drowsiness; impairment of motor skills.	1	2
Insulin	Concurrent use of Ethanol and Insulin may result in increased hypoglycemia.	1	2
Insulin lispro	Concurrent use of Ethanol and Insulin lispro may result in increased hypoglycemia.	1	2
Isoniazid	Concurrent use of Ethanol and Isoniazid may result in decreased isoniazid concentrations and disulfiram-like reactions.	2	1
Isotretinoin	Concurrent use of Ethanol and Isotretinoin may result in a disulfiram-like reaction.	1	1
Kava	Concurrent use of Kava and Ethanol may result in increased central nervous system depression.	1	2
Ketoconazole	Concurrent use of Ethanol and Ketoconazole may result in disulfiram-like reactions (flushing, vomiting, increased respiratory rate, tachycardia).	1	1
Lofepramine	Concurrent use of Ethanol and Lofepramine may result in enhanced drowsiness; impairment of motor skills.	1	2
Lorazepam	Concurrent use of Ethanol and Lorazepam may result in increased sedation.	1	2
Meperidine	Concurrent use of Meperidine and Ethanol may result in increased sedation.	1	2
Mephobarbital	Concurrent use of Mephobarbital and Ethanol may result in excessive CNS depression.	1	2
Meprobamate	Concurrent use of Ethanol and Meprobamate may result in increased sedation.	1	2
Mesoridazine	Concurrent use of Mesoridazine and Ethanol may result in increased central nervous system depression and an increased risk of extrapyramidal reactions.	1	2
Metformin	Concurrent use of Metformin and Ethanol may result in an increased risk of lactic acidosis.	2	2
Methadone	Concurrent use of Ethanol and Methadone may result in increased sedation.	1	2
Methohexital	Concurrent use of Methohexital and Ethanol may result in excessive CNS depression.	1	2
Methotrexate	Concurrent use of Ethanol and Methotrexate may result in increased hepatotoxicity.	2	2
Methotrimeprazine	Concurrent use of Methotrimeprazine and Ethanol may result in increased central nervous system depression and an increased risk of extrapyramidal reactions.	1	2
Metronidazole	Concurrent use of Ethanol and Metronidazole may result in disulfiram-like reactions (flushing, increased respiratory rate, tachycardia) or sudden death.	1	1
Mirtazapine	Concurrent use of Mirtazapine and Ethanol may result in psychomotor impairment.	1	2
Morphine	Concurrent use of Ethanol and Morphine may result in increased sedation.	1	2

(Continued on next page)

Product	Interaction	Onset	Severity
Moxalactam	Concurrent use of Ethanol and Moxalactam may result in disulfiram-like reactions.	2	1
Nefazodone	Concurrent use of Ethanol and Nefazodone may result in an increased risk of CNS side effects.	1	3
Nilutamide	Concurrent use of Ethanol and Nilutamide may result in an increased risk of ethanol intolerance (facial flushing, malaise, and hypotension).	1	3
Nitroglycerin	Concurrent use of Ethanol and Nitroglycerin may result in hypotension.	1	2
Nortriptyline	Concurrent use of Ethanol and Nortriptyline may result in enhanced drowsiness; impairment of motor skills.	1	2
Olanzapine	Concurrent use of Olanzapine and Ethanol may result in excessive central nervous system depression.	1	2
Oxycodone	Concurrent use of Ethanol and Oxycodone may result in increased sedation.	1	2
Paraldehyde	Concurrent use of Paraldehyde and Ethanol may result in metabolic acidosis.	2	2
Paroxetine	Concurrent use of Ethanol and Paroxetine may result in an increased risk of impairment of mental and motor skills.	1	3
Pentazocine	Concurrent use of Pentazocine and Ethanol may result in increased sedation.	1	2
Pentobarbital	Concurrent use of Ethanol and Pentobarbital may result in excessive CNS depression.	1	2
Perphenazine	Concurrent use of Perphenazine and Ethanol may result in increased central nervous system depression and an increased risk of extrapyramidal reactions.	1	2
Phenelzine	Concurrent use of Phenelzine and Ethanol may result in hypertensive urgency or emergency.	1	2
Phenobarbital	Concurrent use of Ethanol and Phenobarbital may result in excessive CNS depression.	1	2
Phenytoin	Concurrent use of Phenytoin and Ethanol may result in decreased phenytoin serum concentrations, increased seizure potential, and additive CNS depressant effects.	1	2
Pipotiazine	Concurrent use of Pipotiazine and Ethanol may result in increased central nervous system depression and an increased risk of extrapyramidal reactions.	1	2
Primidone	Concurrent use of Primidone and Ethanol may result in excessive CNS depression.	1	2
Procarbazine	Concurrent use of Ethanol and Procarbazine may result in disulfiram-like reactions and increased sedation.	1	1
Prochlorperazine	Concurrent use of Prochlorperazine and Ethanol may result in increased central nervous system depression and an increased risk of extrapyramidal reactions.	1	2
Promazine	Concurrent use of Promazine and Ethanol may result in increased central nervous system depression and an increased risk of extrapyramidal reactions.	1	2
Propiomazine	Concurrent use of Propiomazine and Ethanol may result in increased central nervous system depression and an increased risk of extrapyramidal reactions.	1	2
Propoxyphene	Concurrent use of Propoxyphene and Ethanol may result in additive central nervous system depressant effects.	1	2
Protriptyline	Concurrent use of Ethanol and Protriptyline may result in enhanced drowsiness; impairment of motor skills.	1	2
Quetiapine	Concurrent use of Quetiapine and Ethanol may result in potentiation of the cognitive and motor effects of alcohol.	1	2
Secobarbital	Concurrent use of Secobarbital and Ethanol may result in excessive CNS depression.	1	2
Sertraline	Concurrent use of Ethanol and Sertraline may result in an increased risk of impairment of mental and motor skills.	1	3

Product	Interaction	Onset	Severity
Sodium oxybate	Concurrent use of Sodium Oxybate and Ethanol may result in increased sedation.	1	2
Sulfamethoxazole	Concurrent use of Ethanol and Cotrimoxazole may result in disulfiram-like reactions (flushing, sweating, palpitations, drowsiness).	1	1
Temazepam	Concurrent use of Ethanol and Temazepam may result in impaired psychomotor functions.	1	2
Thiethylperazine	Concurrent use of Thiethylperazine and Ethanol may result in increased central nervous system depression and an increased risk of extrapyramidal reactions.	1	2
Thiopental	Concurrent use of Thiopental and Ethanol may result in excessive CNS depression.	1	2
Thioridazine	Concurrent use of Thioridazine and Ethanol may result in increased central nervous system depression and an increased risk of extrapyramidal reactions.	1	2
Tizanidine	Concurrent use of Tizanidine and Ethanol may result in an increased risk of tizanidine adverse effects (excessive CNS depression).	1	2
Tolazamide	Concurrent use of Ethanol and Tolazamide may result in prolonged hypoglycemia, disulfiram-like reactions.	1	1
Tolazoline	Concurrent use of Tolazoline and Ethanol may result in disulfiram-like reactions.	2	1
Tolbutamide	Concurrent use of Ethanol and Tolbutamide may result in prolonged hypoglycemia, disulfiram-like reactions.	1	1
Tramadol	Concurrent use of Ethanol and Tramadol may result in an increased risk of excessive CNS depression.	1	2
Tranylcypromine	Concurrent use of Tranylcypromine and Ethanol may result in hypertensive urgency or emergency.	1	2
Triazolam	Concurrent use of Ethanol and Triazolam may result in increased sedation.	1	2
Trifluoperazine	Concurrent use of Trifluoperazine and Ethanol may result in increased central nervous system depression and an increased risk of extrapyramidal reactions.	1	2
Triflupromazine	Concurrent use of Triflupromazine and Ethanol may result in increased central nervous system depression and an increased risk of extrapyramidal reactions.	1	2
Trimethoprim	Concurrent use of Ethanol and Cotrimoxazole may result in disulfiram-like reactions (flushing, sweating, palpitations, drowsiness).	1	1
Trimipramine	Concurrent use of Ethanol and Trimipramine may result in enhanced drowsiness and impairment of motor skills.	1	2
Valerian	Concurrent use of Valerian and Ethanol may result in increased sedation.	1	2
Venlafaxine	Concurrent use of Ethanol and Venlafaxine may result in an increased risk of CNS effects.	1	3
Verapamil	Concurrent use of Ethanol and Verapamil may result in enhanced ethanol intoxication (impaired psychomotor functioning).	1	2
Warfarin	Concurrent use of Ethanol and Warfarin may result in increased or decreased international normalized ratio (INR) or prothrombin time.	2	2
Zaleplon	Concurrent use of Zaleplon and Ethanol may result in impaired psychomotor functions.	1	2
Zolpidem	Concurrent use of Ethanol and Zolpidem may result in increased sedation.	1	2

Onset: 1 = Rapid (within 24 hours)
2 = Delayed (after 24 hours)
Severity: 1 = Major (possible life-threatening or potential permanent damage)
2 = Moderate (may exacerbate patient's condition)
3 = Minor (little if any clinical effect)
Reprinted with permission from *The Drug Topics Red Book*. Thomson Medical Economics: Montvale, NJ, 2002.

Drug–Tobacco Interactions

Product	Interaction	Onset	Severity
Fluvoxamine	Concurrent use of Fluvoxamine and Tobacco may result in increased fluvoxamine metabolism.	2	3
Imipramine	Concurrent use of Imipramine and Tobacco may result in decreased imipramine concentrations.	2	2
Nortriptyline	Concurrent use of Nortriptyline and Tobacco may result in decreased nortriptyline concentrations.	2	2
Oral contraceptives	Concurrent use of Oral Contraceptives, Combination and Tobacco may result in an increased risk of cardiovascular disease.	2	3
Pentazocine	Concurrent use of Pentazocine and Tobacco may result in decreased pentazocine concentrations.	2	2
Propoxyphene	Concurrent use of Propoxyphene and Tobacco may result in decreased propoxyphene concentrations.	2	2
Theophylline	Concurrent use of Theophylline and Tobacco may result in decreased theophylline concentrations.	2	2
Tolbutamide	Concurrent use of Tolbutamide and Tobacco may result in decreased tolbutamide concentrations.	2	2
Warfarin	Concurrent use of Tobacco and Warfarin may result in increased or decreased international normalized ratio (INR) or prothrombin time.	2	2

Onset: 1 = Rapid (within 24 hours)
               2 = Delayed (after 24 hours)
Severity: 1 = Major (possible life-threatening or potential permanent damage)
               2 = Moderate (may exacerbate patient's condition)
               3 = Minor (little if any clinical effect)
Reprinted with permission from *The Drug Topics Red Book*. Thomson Medical Economics: Montvale, NJ, 2002.

Use-In-Pregnancy Ratings

The U.S. Food & Drug Administration's Use-in-Pregnancy rating system weighs the degree to which available information has ruled out risk to the fetus against the drug's potential benefit to the patient. Following is a listing of drugs (by generic name) for which ratings are available.

X

CONTRAINDICATED IN PREGNANCY

Studies in animals or humans, or investigational or post-marketing reports, have demonstrated fetal risk which clearly outweighs any possible benefit to the patient.

Acitretin
Atorvastatin Calcium
Bicalutamide
Biperiden Hydrochloride
Cerivastatin Sodium
Clomiphene Citrate
Danazol
Demecarium Bromide
Desogestrel/Ethinyl Estradiol
Diclofenac Sodium/Misoprostol

Dienestrol
Dihydroergotamine Mesylate
Estazolam
Estradiol
Estrogens, Conjugated
Estrogens, Conjugated/
    Medroxyprogesterone Acetate
Estrogens, Esterified
Estrogens, Esterified/
    Methyltestosterone
Estropipate
Ethinyl Estradiol
Ethinyl Estradiol/Ethynodiol
    Diacetate
Ethinyl Estradiol/Levonorgestrel
Ethinyl Estradiol/Norethindrone
Ethinyl Estradiol/Norethindrone
    Acetate
Ethinyl Estradiol/Norgestimate
Ethinyl Estradiol/Norgestrel
Finasteride
Fluorouracil

Fluvastatin Sodium
Follitropin Alpha
Follitropin Beta
Gonadotropin, Chorionic
    (Profasi)
Goserelin Acetate
Interferon Alfa-2B/Ribavirin
Isotretinoin
Leflunomide
Leuprolide Acetate
Levonorgestrel
Lovastatin
Medroxyprogesterone Acetate
Megestrol Acetate
Menotropins
Mestranol/Norethindrone
Methyltestosterone
Misoprostol
Nafarelin Acetate
Norethindrone
Norethindrone Acetate
Norgestrel

Oxandrolone
Oxymetholone
Plicamycin
Pravastatin Sodium
Raloxifene Hydrochloride
Ribavirin
Simvastatin
Stanozolol
Tazarotene
Testosterone
Testosterone Enanthate
Thalidomide
Triazolam
Urofollitropin
Vitamin A Palmitate
Warfarin Sodium
Yohimbine Hydrochloride

D

POSITIVE EVIDENCE OF RISK

*Investigational or postmarketing
data show risk to the fetus.
Nevertheless, potential benefits
may outweigh the potential
risk.*

Alitretinoin
Alprazolam
Altretamine
Amiodarone Hydrochloride
Amlodipine Besylate/Benazepril
   Hydrochloride*
Anastrozole
Atenolol
Atenolol/Chlorthalidone
Azathioprine
Azathioprine Sodium
Benazepril Hydrochloride*
Benazepril Hydrochloride/
   Hydrochlorothiazide*
Busulfan
Candesartan Cilexetil*
Capecitabine
Captopril*
Carbamazepine
Carboplatin
Carmustine
Cladribine
Clonazepam
Cytarabine Liposome
Dactinomycin
Daunorubicin Citrate Liposome
Daunorubicin Hydrochloride
Demeclocycline Hydrochloride
Divalproex Sodium
Docetaxel
Doxorubicin Hydrochloride
Doxorubicin Hydrochloride
   Liposome

Doxycycline Calcium
Doxycycline Hyclate
Doxycycline Monohydrate
Enalapril Maleate*
Enalapril Maleate/Felodipine*
Enalapril Maleate/
   Hydrochlorothiazide
Enalaprilat*
Floxuridine
Fludarabine Phosphate
Flutamide
Fosinopril Sodium*
Fosphenytoin Sodium
Gemcitabine Hydrochloride
Hydrochlorothiazide/Irbesartan*
Hydrochlorothiazide/Lisinopril*
Hydrochlorothiazide/Losartan
   Potassium*
Hydrochlorothiazide/Moexipril
   Hydrochloride*
Hydrochlorothiazide/Valsartan*
Idarubicin Hydrochloride
Ifosfamide
Irbesartan*
Lisinopril*
Lithium Carbonate
Lithium Citrate
Lorazepam
Losartan Potassium*
Mechlorethamine Hydrochloride
Melphalan
Mephobarbital
Mercaptopurine
Methimazole
Midazolam Hydrochloride
Minocycline Hydrochloride
Mitoxantrone Hydrochloride
Moexipril Hydrochloride*
Neomycin Sulfate/Polymyxin B
   Sulfate
Nicotine
Paclitaxel
Pentobarbital Sodium
Pentostatin
Perindopril Erbumine*
Potassium Iodide
Procarbazine Hydrochloride
Quinapril Hydrochloride*
Ramipril*
Streptomycin Sulfate
Tamoxifen Citrate
Telmisartan
Thioguanine
Thiotepa
Tobramycin (Inhalation)
Tobramycin Sulfate
Topotecan Hydrochloride
Toremifene Citrate
Trandolapril*
Trandolapril/Verapamil
   Hydrochloride*

Tretinoin (Oral)
Valproate Sodium
Valproic Acid
Valsartan*
Vinblastine Sulfate
Vincristine Sulfate
Vinorelbine Tartrate

C

RISK CANNOT BE
RULED OUT

*Human studies are lacking, and
animal studies are either
positive for risk or are lacking
as well. However, potential
benefits may outweigh the
potential risk.*

Abacavir Sulfate
Abciximab
Acetaminophen/Butalbital
Acetaminophen/Butalbital/
   Caffeine
Acetaminophen/Caffeine/
   Chlorpheniramine Maleate/
   Hydrocodone Bitartrate/
   Phenylephrine Hydrochloride
Acetaminophen/Codeine
   Phosphate
Acetaminophen/Hydrocodone
   Bitartrate
Acetaminophen/Oxycodone
   Hydrochloride
Acetaminophen/Pentazocine
   Hydrochloride
Acetazolamide
Acetic Acid/Oxyquinoline
   Sulfate/Ricinoleic Acid
Acyclovir (Topical)
Adapalene
Adenosine
Alatrofloxacin Mesylate
Albendazole
Albumin, Human
Albuterol
Albuterol Sulfate
Albuterol Sulfate/Ipratropium
   Bromide
Alclometasone Dipropionate
Aldesleukin
Alendronate Sodium
Allopurinol Sodium
Alprostadil
Alteplase, Recombinant
Amantadine Hydrochloride
Amifostine
Aminohippurate Sodium
Aminosalicylic Acid
(Continued on next page)

Amlodipine Besylate
Amlodipine Besylate/Benazepril
Hydrochloride*
Amoxicillin/Clarithromycin/
Lansoprazole
Amphetamine &
Dextroamphetamine Mixture
Amprenavir
Amylase/Cellulase/
Hyoscyamine Sulfate/Lipase/
Phenyltoloxamine Citrate/
Protease
Amylase/Cellulase/Lipase/
Protease
Amylase/Lipase/Protease
Anagrelide Hydrochloride
Antihemophilic Factor IX
Complex (Human)
Antihemophilic Factor IX
Complex (Recombinant)
Antihemophilic Factor VIIa
(Recombinant)
Antihemophilic Factor VIII
(Human)
Antihemophilic Factor VIII
(Human)/Von Willebrand
Factor Complex (Human)
Antihemophilic Factor VIII
(Recombinant)
Antihemophilic Factor VIII:c
(Human)
Anti-Inhibitor Coagulant
Complex
Antipyrine/Benzocaine
Anti-Thymocyte Globulin
Antivenin (Latrodectus Mactans)
Apraclonidine Hydrochloride
Asparaginase
Aspirin/Carisoprodol
Aspirin/Carisoprodol/Codeine
Phosphate
Aspirin/Methocarbamol
Atovaquone
Atropine Sulfate/Benzoic Acid/
Hyoscyamine Sulfate/
Methenamine/Methylene
Blue/Phenyl Salicylate
Atropine Sulfate/Difenoxin
Hydrochloride
Atropine Sulfate/Diphenoxylate
Hydrochloride
Atropine Sulfate/Hyoscyamine
Sulfate/Phenobarbital/
Scopolamine Hydrobromide
Azelastine Hydrochloride
Bacillus of Calmette & Guerin,
Live
Becaplermin
Beclomethasone Dipropionate
Beclomethasone Dipropionate
Monohydrate

Benazepril Hydrochloride*
Benazepril Hydrochloride/
Hydrochlorothiazide*
Bendroflumethiazide/Nadolol
Benzocaine
Benzonatate
Benzoyl Peroxide
Benzoyl Peroxide/
Erythromycin
Bepridil Hydrochloride
Betamethasone Dipropionate,
Augmented
Betamethasone Dipropionate/
Clotrimazole
Betaxolol Hydrochloride
Bethanechol Chloride
Biperiden Lactate
Bisoprolol Fumarate
Bisoprolol Fumarate/
Hydrochlorothiazide
Botulinum Toxin Type A
Brinzolamide
Budesonide
Bupivacaine Hydrochloride
Bupivacaine Hydrochloride/
Epinephrine Bitartrate
Buprenorphine Hydrochloride
Butabarbital/Hyoscyamine
Hydrobromide/
Phenazopyridine
Hydrochloride
Butorphanol Tartrate
Calcitonin, Salmon
Calcitriol
Calcium Acetate
Candesartan Cilexetil*
Captopril*
Carbachol
Carbetapentane Tannate/
Chlorpheniramine Tannate/
Ephedrine Tannate/
Phenylephrine Tannate
Carbetapentane Tannate/
Chlorpheniramine Tannate/
Phenylephrine Tannate
Carbidopa/Levodopa
Carvedilol
Celecoxib
Chloramphenicol
Chloroprocaine Hydrochloride
Chlorothiazide
Chlorothiazide Sodium
Chlorothiazide/Methyldopa
Chloroxine
Chlorpheniramine Maleate/
Methscopolamine Nitrate/
Phenylephrine Hydrochloride
Chlorpheniramine Maleate/
Pseudoephedrine
Hydrochloride

Chlorpheniramine Polistirex/
Hydrocodone Polistirex
Chlorpheniramine Tannate/
Phenylephrine Tannate/
Pyrilamine Tannate
Chlorpropamide
Chlorthalidone/Clonidine
Hydrochloride
Choline Magnesium Trisalicylate
Cidofovir
Cilastatin Sodium/Imipenem
Cilostazol
Ciprofloxacin
Ciprofloxacin Hydrochloride
Ciprofloxacin Hydrochloride/
Hydrocortisone
Citalopram Hydrobromide
Clarithromycin
Clobetasol Propionate
Clofibrate
Clonidine
Clonidine Hydrochloride
Clotrimazole (Oral)
Codeine Phosphate/Guaifenesin
Codeine Phosphate/
Phenylephrine Hydrochloride/
Promethazine Hydrochloride
Codeine Phosphate/
Promethazine Hydrochloride
Colistimethate Sodium
Corticorelin Ovine Triflutate
Corticotropin, Repository
Cosyntropin
Crotamiton
Cyclosporine
Cytomegalovirus Immune
Globulin Intravenous, Human
Dacarbazine
Daclizumab
Dantrolene Sodium
Dapsone
Deferoxamine Mesylate
Delavirdine Mesylate
Denileukin Diftitox
Desonide
Desoximetasone
Dexamethasone Sodium
Phosphate
Dexamethasone Sodium
Phosphate/Neomycin Sulfate
Dexamethasone/Neomycin
Sulfate/Polymyxin B Sulfate
Dexamethasone/Tobramycin
Dexrazoxane
Dextroamphetamine Sulfate
Dextromethorphan
Hydrobromide/Guaifenesin
Dextromethorphan
Hydrobromide/Guaifenesin/
Phenylpropanolamine
Hydrochloride

Dextromethorphan Hydrobromide/Promethazine Hydrochloride
Dextrose/Milrinone Lactate
Dextrose/Vancomycin Hydrochloride
Dichlorphenamide
Diflorasone Diacetate
Diflunisal
Digoxin
Digoxin Immune Fab (Ovine)
Diltiazem Hydrochloride
Dinoprostone
Diphtheria Toxoid/Haemophilus B Conjugate Vaccine/Pertussis Vaccine/Tetanus Toxoid
Diphtheria Toxoid/Pertussis Vaccine, Acellular/Tetanus Toxoid
Diphtheria Toxoid/Tetanus Toxoid
Dirithromycin
Disopyramide Phosphate
Donepezil Hydrochloride
Dorzolamide Hydrochloride
Dorzolamide Hydrochloride/Timolol Maleate
Doxazosin Mesylate
Dronabinol
Dyphylline
Dyphylline/Guaifenesin
Efavirenz
Enalapril Maleate*
Enalapril Maleate/Felodipine*
Enalapril Maleate/Hydrochlorothiazide
Enalaprilat*
Epinephrine
Epinephrine Hydrochloride
Epoetin Alfa
Erythromycin Ethylsuccinate/Sulfisoxazole Acetyl
Esmolol Hydrochloride
Ethiodized Oil
Ethionamide
Etidronate Disodium
Etodolac
Felbamate
Felodipine
Fenofibrate
Fentanyl
Fentanyl Citrate
Ferrous Fumarate/Folic Acid/Intrinsic Factor/Vitamin B12/Vitamin C
Ferrous Fumarate/Folic Acid/Vitamins, Multi
Fexofenadine Hydrochloride
Fexofenadine Hydrochloride/Pseudoephedrine

Hydrochloride
Filgrastim (G-CSF)
Flecainide Acetate
Fluconazole
Flucytosine
Flumazenil
Flunisolide
Flucinolone Acetonide
Fluocinonide
Fluorometholone
Fluorometholone Acetate
Fluorometholone/Sulfacetamide Sodium
Flurandrenolide
Fluticasone Propionate
Fluvoxamine Maleate
Foscarnet Sodium
Fosinopril Sodium*
Furosemide
Gabapentin
Ganciclovir
Ganciclovir Sodium
Gemfibrozil
Gentamicin Sulfate
Glimepiride
Glipizide
Globulin, Immune
Glyburide
Gonadotropin, Chorionic (Novarel)
Guaifenesin
Guaifenesin/Hydrocodone Bitartrate
Guaifenesin/Hydrocodone Bitartrate/Pseudoephedrine Hydrochloride
Guaifenesin/Pseudoephedrine Hydrochloride (Duratuss, Zephrex)
Haemophilus B Conjugate Vaccine
Haemophilus B Conjugate Vaccine/Hepatitis B, Recombinant Vaccine
Halcinonide
Haloperidol Decanoate
Halothane
Hemin
Heparin Sodium
Hepatitis A Vaccine, Inactivated
Hepatitis B Immune Globulin
Hepatitis B Vaccine–Recombinant
Hexachlorophene
Homatropine Methylbromide/Hydrocodone Bitartrate
Homeopathic Product
Hydrochlorothiazide/Irbesartan*
Hydrochlorothiazide/Lisinopril*
Hydrochlorothiazide/Losartan Potassium*

Hydrochlorothiazide/Methyldopa
Hydrochlorothiazide/Metoprolol Tartrate
Hydrochlorothiazide/Moexipril Hydrochloride*
Hydrochlorothiazide/Propranolol Hydrochloride
Hydrochlorothiazide/Spironolactone
Hydrochlorothiazide/Timolol Maleate
Hydrochlorothiazide/Triamterene
Hydrochlorothiazide/Valsartan*
Hydrocodone Bitartrate/Ibuprofen
Hydrocortisone
Hydrocortisone Acetate
Hydrocortisone Acetate/Neomycin Sulfate/Polymyxin B Sulfate
Hydrocortisone Acetate/Pramoxine Hydrochloride
Hydrocortisone Butyrate
Hydrocortisone Probutate
Hydrocortisone Valerate
Hydrocortisone/Iodoquinol
Hydrocortisone/Neomycin Sulfate/Polymyxin B Sulfate
Hydroflumethiazide
Hydromorphone Hydrochloride
Hydroquinone
Hyoscyamine
Hyoscyamine Sulfate
Ibutilide Fumarate
Imiglucerase
Indinavir Sulfate
Indocyanine Green
Influenza Virus Vaccine (Subvirion)
Influenza Virus Vaccine (Whole-Virus)
Interferon Alfa-2A
Interferon Alfa-2B
Interferon Alfacon-1
Interferon Alfa-N3
Interferon Beta-1A
Interferon Beta-1B
Interferon Gamma-1B
Irbesartan*
Iron Dextran
Isoniazid/Pyrazinamide/Rifampin
Isosorbide Dinitrate
Isosorbide Mononitrate (Ismo)
Isradipine
Itraconazole
Ivermectin

(Continued on next page)

Japanese Encephalitis Virus
  Vaccine
Ketoconazole
Ketorolac Tromethamine
Labetalol Hydrochloride
Lamivudine
Lamivudine/Zidovudine
Lamotrigine
Latanoprost
Levalbuterol Hydrochloride
Levamisole Hydrochloride
Levofloxacin
Levorphanol Tartrate
Lisinopril*
Losartan Potassium*
Lyme Disease Vaccine
  (Recombinant OSPA)
Mafenide Acetate
Measles/Mumps/Rubella
  Vaccine
Mebendazole
Mefenamic Acid
Mefloquine Hydrochloride
Meningitis Vaccine
Mepivacaine Hydrochloride
Metaproterenol Sulfate
Metaraminol Bitartrate
Methamphetamine
  Hydrochloride
Methenamine Mandelate/
  Sodium Acid Phosphate
Methocarbamol
Methoxsalen
Metoprolol Succinate
Metoprolol Tartrate
Metyrosine
Mexiletine Hydrochloride
Midodrine Hydrochloride
Milrinone Lactate
Mirtazapine
Modafinil
Moexipril Hydrochloride*
Mometasone Furoate
Monobenzone
Morphine Sulfate
Mumps Virus Vaccine
Muromonab-Cd3
Mycophenolate Mofetil
Mycophenolate Mofetil
  Hydrochloride
Nabumetone
Nadolol
Nalidixic Acid
Naloxone Hydrochloride/
  Pentazocine Hydrochloride
Naphazoline Hydrochloride
Naratriptan Hydrochloride
Natamycin
Nefazodone Hydrochloride
Neostigmine Methylsulfate
Niacin

Nicardipine Hydrochloride
Nifedipine
Nilutamide
Nimodipine
Nisoldipine
Nitroglycerin
Norfloxacin
Nystatin
Ofloxacin
Olanzapine
Olopatadine Hydrochloride
Olsalazine Sodium
Omeprazole
Oprelvekin
Orphenadrine Citrate
Oxaprozin
Oxymorphone Hydrochloride
Palivizumab
Pamidronate Disodium
Pancrelipase
Paricalcitol
Paroxetine Hydrochloride
Pegademase Bovine
Pegaspargase
Penbutolol Sulfate
Pentoxifylline
Perindopril Erbumine*
Phentermine Hydrochloride
Phenylephrine Hydrochloride
Phenylephrine Hydrochloride/
  Promethazine Hydrochloride
Phytonadione
Pilocarpine Hydrochloride
Pimozide
Pioglitazone Hydrochloride
Pirbuterol Acetate
Piroxicam
Plasma Protein Fraction
Pneumococcal Vaccine
Podofilox
Polio Vaccine, Inactivated
Polyethylene Glycol
Polyethylene Glycol/
  Potassium Chloride/
  Sodium
Polyethylene Glycol/Potassium
  Chloride/Sodium
  Bicarbonate/Sodium
  Chloride/Sodium Sulfate
Polymyxin B Sulfate/
  Trimethoprim Sulfate
Polythiazide/Prazosin
  Hydrochloride
Potassium Acid Phosphate
Potassium Chloride
Potassium Citrate
Potassium Phosphate/Dibasic
  Sodium Phosphate/Monobasic
  Sodium Phosphate
Potassium Phosphate/Sodium
  Phosphate

Pralidoxime Chloride
Pramipexole Dihydrochloride
Prazosin Hydrochloride
Prednicarbate
Prednisolone Acetate
Prednisolone Acetate/
  Sulfacetamide Sodium
Prednisolone Sodium Phosphate
Procainamide Hydrochloride
Promethazine Hydrochloride
Propafenone Hydrochloride
Proparacaine Hydrochloride
Propranolol Hydrochloride
Protamine Sulfate
Proteinase Inhibitor (Human),
  Alpha 1
Protirelin
Pyrazinamide
Pyrimethamine
Quetiapine Fumarate
Quinapril Hydrochloride*
Quinidine Gluconate
Quinidine Sulfate
Rabies Immune Globulin
Rabies Vaccine
Ramipril*
Repaglinide
Reteplase, Recombinant
Rho (D) Immune Globulin
Rifampin
Rifapentine
Riluzole
Rimantadine Hydrochloride
Rimexolone
Risedronate Sodium
Risperidone
Rituximab
Rizatriptan Benzoate
Rocuronium Bromide
Rofecoxib
Ropinirole Hydrochloride
Rosiglitazone Maleate
Rubella Virus Vaccine
Rubeola Virus Vaccine
Salicylsalicylic Acid
Salmeterol Xinafoate
Sargramostim
Scopolamine
Selegiline Hydrochloride
Sermorelin Acetate
Sertraline Hydrochloride
Sevelamer Hydrochloride
Sibutramine Hydrochloride
Sodium Polystyrene Sulfonate
Somatrem
Somatropin, E-Coli Derived
Spironolactone
Stavudine
Streptokinase
Succimer
Succinylcholine Chloride

Sulconazole Nitrate
Sulfabenzamide/Sulfacetamide/
  Sulfathiazole
Sulfacetamide Sodium
Sulfacetamide Sodium/Sulfur
Sulfamethoxazole/Trimethoprim
Sulfanilamide
Sumatriptan
Sumatriptan Succinate
Tacrine Hydrochloride
Tacrolimus
Telmisartan*
Terazosin Hydrochloride
Terconazole
Tetanus Immune Globulin
Tetanus Toxoid
Theophylline
Thiabendazole
Thrombin
Thyrotropin Alfa
Tiagabine Hydrochloride
Tiludronate Disodium
Timolol Maleate
Tizanidine Hydrochloride
Tocainide Hydrochloride
Tolcapone
Tolmetin Sodium
Tolterodine Tartrate
Topiramate
Tramadol Hydrochloride
Trandolapril*
Trandolapril/Verapamil
  Hydrochloride*
Tretinoin (Topical)
Triamcinolone Acetonide
Triamterene
Trientine Hydrochloride
Triethanolamine Polypeptide
  Oleate
Trifluridine
Trimethoprim
Trimipramine Maleate
Trovafloxacin Mesylate
Tuberculin
Typhoid Vaccine
Typhoid Vi Polysaccharide
  Vaccine
Valrubicin
Valsartan*
Varicella Virus Vaccine
Vecuronium Bromide
Venlafaxine Hydrochloride
Verapamil Hydrochloride
Vitamin B12
Yellow Fever Vaccine
Zalcitabine
Zaleplon
Zidovudine
Zileuton
Zolmitriptan

B

NO EVIDENCE OF RISK IN HUMANS

Either animal findings show risk while human findings do not, or, if no adequate human studies have been done, animal findings are negative.

Acarbose
Acebutolol Hydrochloride
Acrivastine/Pseudoephedrine
  Hydrochloride
Acyclovir (Oral)
Acyclovir Sodium
Amiloride Hydrochloride
Amiloride Hydrochloride/
  Hydrochlorothiazide
Amlexanox
Amoxicillin
Amoxicillin/Clavulanate
  Potassium
Amphotericin B Lipid Complex
Amphotericin B Liposome
Ampicillin Sodium/Sulbactam
  Sodium
Amylase/Lipase/Protease
  (Pancrease)
Antithrombin III (Human)
Aprotinin
Azelaic Acid
Azithromycin Dihydrate
Aztreonam
Basiliximab
Brimonidine Tartrate
Bupropion Hydrochloride
Butenafine Hydrochloride
Cabergoline
Carbenicillin Indanyl Sodium
Cefaclor
Cefadroxil
Cefamandole Nafate
Cefazolin Sodium
Cefdinir
Cefepime Hydrochloride
Cefixime
Cefoperazone Sodium
Cefotaxime Sodium
Cefotetan Disodium
Cefoxitin Sodium
Cefpodoxime Proxetil
Cefprozil
Ceftazidime
Ceftazidime Sodium
Ceftibuten
Ceftizoxime Sodium
Ceftriaxone Sodium
Cefuroxime Axetil
Cefuroxime Sodium

Cephalexin
Cetirizine Hydrochloride
Chlorhexidine Gluconate
Ciclopirox Olamine
Cimetidine
Cimetidine Hydrochloride
Clavulanate Potassium/
  Ticarcillin Disodium
Clindamycin Hydrochloride
Clindamycin Phosphate
Clopidogrel Bisulfate
Clotrimazole (Topical)
Clozapine
Cromolyn Sodium
Cyclobenzaprine Hydrochloride
Cyproheptadine Hydrochloride
Dalteparin Sodium
Danaparoid Sodium
Desflurane
Desmopressin Acetate
Diclofenac Potassium
Diclofenac Sodium
Didanosine
Diphenhydramine
  Hydrochloride
Dipyridamole
Dobutamine Hydrochloride
Dolasetron Mesylate
Dornase Alpha
Doxapram Hydrochloride
Edetate Calcium Disodium
Emedastine Difumarate
Enoxaparin Sodium
Epinephrine/Lidocaine
  Hydrochloride
Epoprostenol Sodium
Eptifibatide
Erythromycin
Erythromycin Ethylsuccinate
Erythromycin Stearate
Etanercept
Ethacrynate Sodium
Ethacrynic Acid
Etidocaine Hydrochloride
Famotidine
Fenoldopam Mesylate
Ferric Sodium Gluconate
Flavoxate Hydrochloride
Fosfomycin Tromethamine
Glatiramer Acetate
Glucagon Hydrochloride
Glycopyrrolate
Gonadorelin Hydrochloride
Guaifenesin/Pseudoephedrine
  Hydrochloride (Guaifed)
Guanfacine Hydrochloride
Hydrochlorothiazide
Ibuprofen
Imiquimod
(Continued on next page)

Indapamide
Infliximab
Insulin Lispro, Human
Ipratropium Bromide
Isosorbide Mononitrate
(Monoket, Imdur)
Ketoprofen
Lactulose
Lansoprazole
Lepirudin
Levocarnitine
Lidocaine
Lidocaine Hydrochloride
Lidocaine/Prilocaine
Lindane
Lodoxamide Tromethamine
Loracarbef
Loratadine
Loratadine/Pseudoephedrine
Sulfate
Malathion
Meclizine Hydrochloride
Meropenem
Mesalamine
Metformin Hydrochloride
Methohexital Sodium
Methyldopa
Metoclopramide Hydrochloride
Metolazone
Metronidazole
Metronidazole Hydrochloride
Miglitol
Montelukast Sodium
Mupirocin
Mupirocin Calcium
Naftifine Hydrochloride

Nalbuphine Hydrochloride
Nalmefene Hydrochloride
Naloxone Hydrochloride
Naproxen
Naproxen Sodium
Nelfinavir Mesylate
Nitrofurantoin, Macrocrystals
Nitrofurantoin, Macrocrystals/
Nitrofurantoin Monohydrate
Nizatidine
Octreotide Acetate
Ondansetron
Ondansetron Hydrochloride
Orlistat
Oxiconazole Nitrate
Oxybutynin Chloride
Oxycodone Hydrochloride
Pemoline
Penicillin G Benzathine
Penicillin G Benzathine/
Penicillin G Procaine
Penicillin G Potassium
Pentosan Polysulfate Sodium
Pergolide Mesylate
Permethrin
Piperacillin Sodium
Piperacillin Sodium/
Tazobactam Sodium
Praziquantel
Progesterone
Propofol
Psyllium
Ranitidine Hydrochloride
Rifabutin
Ritonavir
Ropivacaine Hydrochloride

Saquinavir
Saquinavir Mesylate
Sildenafil Citrate
Silver Sulfadiazine
Sodium Fluoride
Somatropin, E-Coli Derived
(Genotropin)
Sotalol Hydrochloride
Sucralfate
Sulfasalazine
Tamsulosin Hydrochloride
Terbinafine Hydrochloride
Terbutaline Sulfate
Ticlopidine Hydrochloride
Tirofiban Hydrochloride
Tobramycin (Ophthalmic)
Torsemide
Trastuzumab
Ursodiol
Valacyclovir Hydrochloride
Vancomycin Hydrochloride
Zafirlukast
Zolpidem Tartrate

A

**CONTROLLED STUDIES
SHOW NO RISK**

*Adequate, well-controlled
studies in pregnant women
have failed to demonstrate risk
to the fetus.*
Levothyroxine Sodium
Liothyronine Sodium

---

* Category C or D depending on the trimester the drug is given.
Reprinted with permission from *The Drug Topics Red Book.* Thomson Medical Economics: Montvale, NJ, 2002.

Drugs Excreted in Breast Milk

The following is a selection of drug products that can be excreted in breast milk. The list is not comprehensive. Generics and alternate brands of some products may exist. When recommending drugs to pregnant or nursing patients, always check product labeling for specific precautions.

Accolate	Alesse	Asacol	Azulfidine	Cafergot
Accuretic	Alfenta	Astramorph/PF	Bactramycin	Calan
Achromycin	Aloprim	Ativan	Bactrim	Capoten
Actiq	Altace	A/T/S	Benadryl	Capozide
Adalat	Ambien	Augmentin	Bentyl	Captopril
Adderall	Anaprox	Avalide	Betapace	Carbatrol
Aggrenox	Ancef	AVC	Bicillin	Cardizem
Aldactazide	Androderm	Axid	Blocadren	Cataflam
Aldactone	Apresoline	Axocet	Brethine	Catapres
Aldomet	Aralen	Azactam	Brevicon	Catapres-TTS
Aldoril	Arthrotec	Azathioprine	Brontex	Ceclor

Cefizox
Cefobid
Cefotan
Ceftin
Celexa
Ceptaz
Cerebyx
Ceredase
Cipro
Claforan
Claritin
Claritin-D
Cleocin
Clorpres
Clozaril
Codeine
CombiPatch
Combipres
Combivir
Compazine
Cordarone
Corgard
Cortisporin
Cortone
Corzide
Cosopt
Coumadin
Covera-HS
Crinone
Cystospaz
Cystospaz-M
Cytotec
Cytoxan
Dalalone D.P.
Dapsone
Daraprim
Darvon
Darvon-N
Decadron
Decadron-LA
Deconsal II
Demerol
Demulen
Depacon
Depakene
Depakote
Depo-Provera
Desogen
Desoxyn
Desyrel
Dexedrine
DextroStat
D.H.E. 45
Diabinese
Diastat
Diflucan
Dilacor
Dilantin
Dilantin-125
Dilaudid
Dilaudid-HP
Diovan

Diprivan
Disalcid
Diucardin
Diuril
Dolobid
Dolophine
Doral
Doryx
Droxia
Duraclon
Duragesic
Duramorph
Duratuss
Duricef
Dyazide
Dyrenium
E.E.S.
EC-Naprosyn
Ecotrin
Effexor
Elavil
EMLA
E-Mycin
Enduron
Equanil
ERYC
EryPed
Ery-Tab
Erythrocin
Erythromycin
Esgic-plus
Eskalith
Estrostep
Ethmozine
Felbatol
Feldene
Fero-Folic
Fiorinal
Flagyl
Florinef
Floxin
Fluorescite
Fortaz
Furosemide
Galzin
Garamycin
Glucophage
Glyset
Guaifed
Guaifed-PD
Halcion
Haldol
Helidac
Hydrocet
Hydrocortone
HydroDIURIL
Iberet-Folic
Ifex
Imitrex
Imuran
Inderal
Inderide

Indocin
INFeD
Inversine
Isoptin
Kadian
Keflex
Keftab
Kefurox
Kefzol
Kerlone
Klonopin
Kutrase
Lamictal
Lamisil
Lamprene
Lanoxicaps
Lanoxin
Lariam
Lescol
Levbid
Levlen
Levlite
Levora
Levothroid
Levoxyl
Levsin
Levsin/SL
Levsinex
Lexxel
Lindane
Lioresal
Lithium
Lithobid
Lo/Ovral
Loestrin
Lomotil
Loniten
Lopressor
Lortab
Lotrel
Ludiomil
Lufyllin
Lufyllin-400
Lufyllin-GG
Luminal
Luvox
Macrobid
Macrodantin
Mandol
Marinol
Maxipime
Maxzide
Maxzide-25
Mefoxin
Mepergan
Meruvax II
Methergine
Methotrexate
MetroCream
MetroGel
MetroLotion
Mexitil

Mezlin
Micronor
Microzide
Midamor
Migranal
Miltown
Minizide
Minocin
Mircette
M-M-R II
Modicon
Moduretic
Monocid
Monodox
Mono-Gesic
Monopril
Morphine
MS Contin
MSIR
Myambutol
Mykrox
Mysoline
Naprelan
Naprosyn
Nascobal
Necon
NegGram
Nembutal
Neoral
Netromycin
Niaspan
Nicotrol
Nizoral
Norco
Nor-QD
Nordette
Norinyl
Noritate
Normodyne
Norpace
Norplant
Novantrone
Nubain
Nucofed
Nydrazid
Oramorph
Oretic
Ortho-Cept
Ortho-Cyclen
Ortho-Novum
Orudis
Ovcon
Ovral
Ovrette
Oxistat
OxyContin
OxyFast
OxyIR
Pacerone
Pamelor
Panlor SS
Paxil

PCE
Pediapred
Pediazole
Pediotic
Pentasa
Pepcid
Periostat
Persantine
Pfizerpen
Phenergan
Phenobarbital
Phrenilin
Pipracil
Plan B
Platinol-AQ
Ponstel
Pravachol
Premphase
Prempro
Prevacid
Preven
PREVPAC
Prinzide
Procanbid
Prograf
Proloprim
Prometrium
Pronestyl
Propofol
Prosed/DS
Provera
Prozac
Pseudoephedrine
Pulmicort
Pyrazinamide
Quibron
Quibron-T
Quibron-T/SR
Quinaglute
Quinidex
Quinine
Reglan
Renese
Requip
Reserpine
Restoril
Retrovir
Ridaura
Rifadin
Rifamate
Rifater
Rimactane
RMS
Robaxisal
Rocaltrol
Rocephin
Roferon A
Roxanol
Roxanol-T
Salflex
Sandimmune

(Continued on next page)

Sansert	Tarka	Tol-Tab	Uni-Dur	Xanax
Seconal	Tavist	Toprol-XL	Uniphyl	Zagam
Sectral	Tazicef	Toradol	Uniretic	Zantac
Sedapap	Tazidime	Trandate	Uroqid-Acid	Zarontin
Semprex-D	Tegretol	Tranxene	Valium	Zaroxolyn
Septra	Tegretol-XR	Tranxene-SD	Vanceril	Zestoretic
Sinequan	Tenoretic	Trental	Vancocin	Ziac
Slo-bid	Tenormin	Trilafon	Vantin	Zinacef
Solganal	Tenuate	Trileptal	Vascor	Zithromax
Soma	Testoderm	Tri-Levlen	Vaseretic	Zoloft
Sonata	Thalitone	Trilisate	Vasotec	Zonalon
Sporanox	Theo-24	Tri-Norinyl	Verelan	Zonegran
Stadol	Theo-Dur	Triostat	Vermox	Zosyn
Stelazine	Theo-X	Triphasil	Versed	Zovia
Streptomycin	Thorazine	Trivora	Vibramycin	Zovirax
Stromectol	Tiazac	Trizivir	Vibra-Tabs	Zyban
Symmetrel	Timolide	Trovan	Vicodin	Zydone
Syn-Rx	Timoptic	Tylenol	Viramune	Zyloprim
Synthroid	Timoptic-XE	Tylenol with	Visken	Zyrtec
Tagamet	Tobi	Codeine	Voltaren	
Tambocor	Tofranil	Ultram	Voltaren-XR	
Tapazole	Tolectin	Unasyn	Wellbutrin	

Reprinted with permission from *The Drug Topics Red Book*. Thomson Medical Economics: Montvale, NJ, 2002.

Dietary Considerations

Potassium and Tyramine Content of Foods
Potassium Content of Foods
High-Potassium Foods

Fruits	Vegetables	Other Foods
Apricot	Artichokes	Bran/Bran products
Avocado	Beans, dried	Coffee (limit 2 cups/day)
Banana	Broccoli	Chocolate
Cantaloupe	Brussels Sprouts	Coconut
Casaba	Celery	Granola
Dates	Escarole	Ice Cream (limit 1 cup/day)
Dried fruits	Endive	Molasses
Figs	Greens (swiss chard, collard,	Nuts/seeds
	dandelion, mustard, beet)	
Honeydew	Kale	Orange flavored pop
Mango	Kohlrabi	Salt substitutes/like salt
Nectarine	Lentils	Snuff/chewing tobacco
Orange	Legumes	Tea (limit 2 cups/day)
Papaya	Lima Beans	
Plums	Mushrooms	
Prunes	Parsnips	
Raisins	Potatoes (french fries, baked, sweet)	
Rhubarb	Salt-free vegetable juice	
Juice of these fruits	Tomatoes	

Low-Potassium Foods

Fruits	Vegetables	Other Foods
Apples	Alfalfa sprouts	Rice
Blackberries	Asparagus	Noodles
Blueberries	Beans, green or wax	Bread & bread products
Boysenberries	Bean sprouts	Cereals
Cherries	Beets	Cake
Cranberries	Cabbage	Cookies

Fruits	Vegetables	Other Foods
Gooseberries	Carrots	Pies (no chocolate or high-potassium fruit)
Grapes	Cauliflower	
Loganberries	Corn	
Mandarin oranges	Cucumber	
Pears	Eggplant	
Pineapple	Lettuce	
Raspberries	Mixed vegetables	
Strawberries	Okra	
Tangerines	Onions	
Watermelon	Parsley	
Juice of these fruits	Peas	
	Radishes	
	Rutabagas	
	Squash (summer, zucchini)	

Tyramine Content of Foods

Food	Allowed	Minimize Intake	Not Allowed
Beverages	Milk, decaffeinated coffee, tea, soda	Chocolate beverage, caffeine-containing drinks, clear spirits	Acidophilus milk, beer, ale, wine, malted beverages
Breads/cereals	All except those containing cheese	None	Cheese bread and crackers
Dairy products	Cottage cheese, farmers or pot cheese, cream cheese, ricotta cheese, all milk, eggs, ice cream, pudding (except chocolate)	Yogurt (limit to 4 oz per day)	All other cheeses (aged cheese, American, Camembert, cheddar, Gouda, gruyere, mozzarella, parmesan, provolone, romano, Roquefort, stilton)
Meat, fish, and poultry	All fresh or frozen	Aged meats, hot dogs, canned fish and meat	Chicken and beef liver, dried and pickled fish, summer or dry sausage, pepperoni, dried meats, meat extracts, bologna, liverwurst
Starches— potatoes/rice	All	None	Soybean (including paste)
Vegetables	All fresh, frozen, canned, or dried vegetable juices except those not allowed	Chili peppers, Chinese pea pods	Fava beans, sauerkraut, pickles, olives, Italian broad beans
Fruit	Fresh, frozen, or canned fruits and fruit juices	Avocado, banana, raspberries, figs	Banana peel extract
Soups	All soups not listed to limit or avoid	Commercially canned soups	Soups which contain broad beans, fava beans, cheese, beer, wine, any made with flavor cubes or meat extract, miso soup
Fats	All except fermented	Sour cream	Packaged gravy
Sweets	Sugar, hard candy, honey, molasses, syrups	Chocolate candies	None
Desserts	Cakes, cookies, gelatin, pastries, sherbets, sorbets	Chocolate desserts	Cheese-filled desserts
Miscellaneous	Salt, nuts, spices, herbs, flavorings, Worcestershire sauce	Soy sauce, peanuts	Brewer's yeast, yeast concentrates, all aged and fermented products, monosodium glutamate, vitamins with Brewer's yeast

NATIONAL AND STATE BOARDS OF PHARMACY CONTACT INFORMATION

This appendix contains the most recent contact information for the national and state boards of pharmacy. A current listing of contact information for state boards of pharmacy is maintained at the National Association of Boards of Pharmacy website, www.napb.com. In addition, contact information for all the pharmacy schools in the United States can be found at the American Association of Colleges of Pharmacy website, www.aacp.org.

NATIONAL ASSOCIATION OF BOARDS OF PHARMACY

Carmen A. Catizone
Executive Director
700 Busse Highway
Park Ridge, IL 60068-2402
847-698-6227, Fax: 847-698-0124
www.nabp.net

STATE BOARDS OF PHARMACY

Alabama
Jerry Moore, RPh
Executive Director
1 Perimeter Park South, Suite 425S
Birmingham, AL 35243
205-967-0130, Fax: 205-967-1009
e-mail: rphbham@bellsouth.net
www.albop.com

Alaska
Barbara Roche
Licensing Examiner
PO Box 110806
Juneau, AK 99811
907-465-2589
www.decd.state.ak.us/occ/ppha.htm

Arizona
Llyn A. Lloyd, RPh
Executive Director
4425 W Olive Avenue, Suite 140
Glendale, AZ 85302
623-463-2727
e-mail: vsevilla@azsbp.com
www.pharmacy.state.az.us

Arkansas
Charles S. Campbell
Executive Director
101 East Capitol Avenue, Suite 218
Little Rock, AR 72201
501-682-0190, Fax: 501-682-0195
e-mail: charlie.campbell@mail.state.ar.us
www.state.ar.us/asbp

California
Patricia Harris
Executive Officer
400 R Street, Suite 4070
Sacramento, CA 95814
916-445-5014, Fax: 916-327-6308
e-mail: patricia_harris@dca.ca.gov
www.pharmacy.ca.gov

Colorado
Susan L. Warren
Program Administrator
1560 Broadway, Suite 1310
Denver, CO 80202
303-984-7750 ext. 313, Fax: 303-894-7764
e-mail: pharmacy@dora.state.co.us
www.dora.state.co.us/pharmacy

Connecticut
Michelle Sylvestre
Drug Control Agent and Board Administrator
State Office Building, Room 110
165 Capitol Avenue
Hartford, CT 06106
860-713-6070, Fax: 860-713-7242
e-mail: michelle.sylvestre@po.state.ct.us
www.ctdrugcontrol.com/rxcommission.htm

Delaware
David W. Dryden, RPh, Esq.
Executive Secretary
PO Box 637
Dover, DE 19903
302-739-4798, Fax: 302-739-3071
e-mail: gbunting@state.de.us
www.professionallicensing.state.de.us

District of Columbia
Graphelia Ramseur
Health Licensing Specialist
825 N Capitol St NE, Room 2224
Washington, DC 20002
202-442-4775, Fax: 202-442-9431
http://dchealth.de.gov/

Florida
John D. Taylor, RPh
Executive Director
4052 Bald Cypress Way, Bin #C04
Tallahassee, FL 32399-3254
850-245-4292
e-mail: mqa_pharmacy@doh.state.fl.us
www.doh.state.fl.us/mqa

Georgia
Anita O. Martin
Executive Director
237 Coliscum Dr
Macon, GA 31217-3858
478-207-1686
www.sos.state.ga.us/plb/pharmacy/

Guam
Teresita Villagomez
Acting Administrator
PO Box 2816
Hagatna, GU 96932
671-735-7406, Fax: 671-735-7413
e-mail: tlgvillagomez@dphss.gcvguam.net

Hawaii
Lee Ann Teshima
Executive Officer
PO Box 3469
Honolulu, HI 96801
808-586-2698, Fax: 808-586-2874
e-mail: pharmacy@dcca.state.hi.us
www.state.hi.us/dcca/pvl/

Idaho
R. K. Markuson, RPh
Executive Director
PO Box 83720
Boise, ID 83720-0067
208-334-2356, Fax: 208-334-3536
www.state.id.us/bop

Illinois
Judy Cullen
Pharmacy Coordinator
Illinois Department of Professional Regulation
320 West Washington Street, Third Floor
Springfield, IL 62786
217-785-0800
www.dpr.state.il.us/

Indiana
Joshua Bolin
Director
402 West Washington Street, Room 041
Indianapolis, IN 46204
317-234-2067
e-mail: hpb4@hpb.state.in.us
www.in.gov/hpb/boards/isbp/

Iowa
Lloyd K. Jessen, RPh, JD
Executive Secretary/Director
400 SW Eighth Street, Suite E
Des Moines, IA 50309-4688
515-281-5944, Fax: 515-281-4609
e-mail: debbie.jorgensen@ibpe.state.ia.us
www.state.ia.us/ibpe

Kansas
Susan Linn
Executive Director
900 Jackson Street SW, Room 513
Landon State Office Building
Topeka, KS 66612-1231
785-296-4056, Fax: 785-296-8420
e-mail: pharmacy@ink.org
www.accesskansas.org/pharmacy

Kentucky
Michael A. Moné, RPh, JD
Executive Director
23 Millcreek Park
Frankfort, KY 40601
502-573-1580, Fax: 502-573-1582
e-mail: pharmacy.board@mail.state.ky.us

Louisiana
Malcolm J. Broussard
Executive Director
5615 Corporate Boulevard, 8E
Baton Rouge, LA 70808
225-925-6496
www.labp.com

Maine
Geraldine Betts
Board Administrator
35 State House Station
Augusta, ME 04333
207-624-8603, Fax: 207-624-8637
Hearing Impaired: 207-624-8563
e-mail: kelly.l.mclaughlin@state.me.us
www.maineprofessionalreg.org

Maryland
LaVerne George Nasea
Executive Director
4201 Patterson Avenue
Baltimore, MD 21215
410-764-4755, Fax: 410-358-6207
e-mail: mdbop@dhmh.state.md.us
www.dhmh.state.md.us/pharmacyboard/

Massachusetts
Charles R. Young
Executive Director
239 Causeway Street
Boston, MA 02113
617-727-9953
e-mail: charles.r.young@state.ma.us
www.state.ma.us/reg/boards/ph

Michigan
Melanie Brim
Licensing Manager
611 West Ottawa, First Floor
PO Box 30670
Lansing, MI 48909-8710
517-373-9102, Fax: 517-373-2179
www.michigan.gov/cis/0,1607,7-154-
    10568_17671_17688-42779--,00.html

Minnesota
David E. Holmstrom, RPh, JD
Executive Director
2829 University Avenue SE, Suite 530
Minneapolis, MN 55414
612-617-2201, Fax: 612-617-2212
e-mail: david.holmstrom@state.mn.us
www.phcybrd.state.mn.us

Mississippi
Leland McDivitt
Executive Director
PO Box 24507
Jackson, MS 39225-4507
601-354-6750, Fax: 601-354-6071
www.mbp.state.ms.us

Missouri
Kevin E. Kinkade, RPh
Executive Director
PO Box 625
Jefferson City, MO 65102
573-751-0091
e-mail: kkinkade@mail.state.mo.us
www.ecodev.state.mo.us/pr/pharmacy

Montana
Rebecca Deschamps, RPh
Executive Director
111 North Jackson
PO Box 200513
Helena, MT 59620-0513
406-841-2356, Fax: 406-841-2343
e-mail: dlibspdha@state.mt.us
http://discoveringmontana.com/dli/bsd/license/
    bsd_boards/pha_board/board_page.htm

Nebraska
Becky Wisell
Executive Secretary
PO Box 94986
Lincoln, NE 68509-4986
402-471-2115
www.hhs.state.ne.us

Nevada
Keith W. MacDonald, RPh
Executive Secretary
555 Double Eagle Court, Suite 1100
Reno, NV 89521
775-850-1440
e-mail: pharmacy@govmail.state.nv.us
http://nvbop.glsuite.us/renewal/glsweb/
    homeframe.aspx

New Hampshire
Paul G. Boisseau, RPh
Executive Director
57 Regional Drive
Concord, NH 03301-8518
603-271-2350, Fax: 603-271-2856
e-mail: nhpharmacy@nhsa.state.nh.us
www.state.nh.us/pharmacy/

New Jersey
Debora C. Whipple
Executive Director
PO Box 45013
Newark, NJ 07101
973-504-6450, Fax: 973-648-3355
e-mail: askconsumeraffairs@dca.lps.state.nj.us

New Mexico
Jerry Montoya
Chief Inspector/Director
1650 University Boulevard NE, Suite 400-B
Albuquerque, NM 87102
505-841-9102, Fax: 505-841-9113
e-mail: joseph.montoya@state.nm.us
www.state.nm.us/pharmacy

New York
Lawrence H. Mokhiber, RPh
Executive Secretary
89 Washington Avenue, Second Floor W
Albany, NY 12234-1000
518-474-3817 ext. 130, Fax: 518-473-6995
www.nysed.gov/prof/pharm.htm

North Carolina
David R. Work, RPh
Executive Director
PO Box 459
Carrboro, NC 27510-0459
919-942-4454, Fax: 919-967-5757
e-mail: drw@ncbop.org
www.ncbop.org

North Dakota
Howard C. Anderson, Jr, RPh
Executive Director
PO Box 1354
Bismarck, ND 58502-1354
701-328-9535, Fax: 701-258-9312
e-mail: ndboph@btinet.net

Ohio
William T. Windsley
Executive Director
77 South High Street, Room 1702
Columbus, OH 43215-6126
614-466-4143, Fax: 614-752-4836
e-mail: exec@bop.state.oh.us
www.state.oh.us/pharmacy/

Oklahoma
Bryan H. Potter, RPh
Executive Director
4545 North Lincoln Boulevard, Suite 112
Oklahoma City, OK 73105-3488
405-521-3815, Fax: 405-521-3758
e-mail: pharmacy@oklaosf.state.ok.us
www.pharmacy.state.ok.us

Oregon
Gary A. Schnabel
Executive Director
State Office Building, Suite 425
800 NE Oregon Street, #9
Portland, OR 97232
503-731-4032, Fax: 503-731-4067
e-mail: pharmacy.board@state.or.us
www.pharmacy.state.or.us

Pennsylvania
Melanie Zimmerman
Executive Secretary
124 Pine Street
PO Box 2649
Harrisburg, PA 17105-2649
717-783-7156, Fax: 717-787-7769
e-mail: pharmacy@pados.dos.state.pa.us
www.dos.state.pa.us/bpoa/phabd/mainpage.htm

Puerto Rico
Magda Bouet Graña
Executive Director
Department of Health, Board of Pharmacy
Call Box 10200
Santurce, PR 00908
787-725-8161, Fax: 787-725-7903

Rhode Island
Catherine A. Cordy
Chief of the Board
3 Capitol Hill, Room 205
Providence, RI 02908
401-222-2837, Fax: 401-222-2158
e-mail: dianet@doh.state.ri.us

South Carolina
LeeAnn Bundrick
Interim Administrator
100 Centerview Drive, Suite 306
Columbia, SC 29211-1927
803-896-4700, Fax: 803-896-4596
e-mail: funderbm@mail.llr.state.sc.us

South Dakota
Dennis M. Jones, RPh
Executive Secretary
4305 South Louise Avenue, Suite 104
Sioux Falls, SD 57106
605-362-2737, Fax: 605-362-2738
e-mail: dennis.jones@state.sd.us
www.state.sd.us/dcr/pharmacy

Tennessee
Kendall M. Lynch
Director
Second Floor, Davy Crockett Tower
500 James Robertson Parkway
Nashville, TN 37243
615-741-2718, Fax: 615-741-2722
e-mail: klynch@mail.state.tn.us
www.state.tn.us/commerce/pharmacy

Texas
Gay Dodson, RPh
Executive Director
333 Guadalupe, Suite 3-600
Box 21
Austin, TX 78701-3942
512-305-8000, Fax: 512-305-8082
e-mail: geninfo@tsbp.state.tx.us
www.tsbp.state.tx.us

Utah
Diana L. Baker
Bureau Director
Division of Occupational and Professional
   Licensing
PO Box 146741
Salt Lake City, UT 84114-6741
801-530-6179, Fax: 801-530-6511
e-mail: dbaker@utah.gov
www.commerce.state.ut.us/dopl/dopl1.htm

Vermont
Peggy Atkins
Board Administrator
26 Terrace Street, Drawer 09
Montpelier, VT 05609-1106
802-828-2875, Fax: 802-828-2465
e-mail: cpreston@sec.state.vt.us
www.vtprofessionals.org

Virgin Islands
Lydia T. Scott
Executive Assistant
Commissioner of Health
Roy L. Schneider Hospital
48 Sugar Estate
St. Thomas, VI 00802
340-774-0117 ext. 5078, Fax: 340-777-4001

Virginia
Elizabeth Scott Russell, RPh
Executive Director
6606 West Broad Street, 4th Floor
Richmond, VA 23230-1717
804-662-9911, Fax: 804-552-9313
e-mail: scotti.russell@dhp.state.va.us
www.dhp.state.va.us/pharmacy/default.htm

Washington
Donald H. Williams, RPh
Executive Director
PO Box 47863
Olympia, WA 98504-7863
360-236-4825, Fax: 360-586-4359
e-mail: don.williams@doh.wa.gov
http://wws2.wa.gov/doh/hpqa-
    licensing/HPS4/Pharmacy/default.htm

West Virginia
William T. Douglass, Jr
Executive Director
232 Capitol Street
Charleston, WV 25301
304-558-0558, Fax: 304-558-0572
e-mail: wdouglass@wvbop.com

Wisconsin
Deanna Zychowski
Director
1400 East Washington
PO Box 8935
Madison, WI 53708
608-266-2812, Fax: 608-267-0644
e-mail: web@drl.state.wi.us
www.state.wi.us/agencies/drl

Wyoming
James T. Carder
Executive Director
1720 South Poplar Street, Suite 4
Casper, WY 82601
307-234-0294, Fax: 307-234-7226
e-mail: wypharmbd@wercs.com
http://pharmacyboard.state.wy.us

BUDGETING FOR DRUG INFORMATION RESOURCES

A. Basic Library

References	Cost*
American Hospital Formulary Service (AHFS) Drug Information	$ 175.00
Drug Facts and Comparisons	$ 180.00
Handbook on Injectable Drugs	$ 170.00
Handbook of Non-Prescription Drugs	$ 129.00
Martindale: The Complete Drug Reference	$ 470.00
Nonprescription Product Therapeutics	$ 107.00
Physicians' Desk Reference	$ 90.00
Remington's Pharmaceutical Sciences	$ 99.00
USP DI (three-volume set)	$ 397.00

B. Additional Resources

References	Cost*
Drug–Drug Interaction	
• *Drug Interactions Analysis & Management*	$ 180.00
• *Drug Interaction Facts*	$ 72.00
• *Evaluations of Drug Interactions*	$ 240.00
Herbal	
• *PDR for Herbal Medicines*	$ 60.00
• *The Review of Natural Products*	$ 80.00
Internal Medicine	
• *Cecil Textbook of Medicine*	$ 139.00
• *Harrison's Principles of Internal Medicine*	$ 125.00
Pediatrics	
• *Pediatric Dosage Handbook*	$ 40.00
• *The Harriet Lane Handbook*	$ 40.00
Pharmacokinetics	
• *Applied Biopharmaceutics and Pharmacokinetics*	$ 55.00
• *Clinical Pharmacokinetics Pocket Reference*	$ 53.00
• *Concepts in Clinical Pharmacokinetics*	$ 79.00
• *Therapeutic Drug Monitoring*	$ 33.00
Pharmacology	
• *Goodman and Gilman's The Pharmacological Basis of Therapeutics*	$ 125.00
Pregnancy/Breast-feeding	
• *Drugs in Pregnancy and Lactation*	$ 140.00
Therapeutics	
• *Applied Therapeutics: The Clinical Use of Drugs*	$ 157.00
• *Pharmacotherapy: A Pathophysiologic Approach*	$ 194.00
• *Textbook of Therapeutics: Drug and Disease Management*	$ 157.00

C. CD-ROM Computer Systems/Programs

	Cost*
AHFS first WEB	$ 2,990.00
Clinical Pharmacology Internet Monograph Service	$ 145.00
Clinical Reference Library (Lexi–Comp) online	$ 350.00
CliniTrend Software	$ 688.00
DataKinetics Software	$ 688.00
eFacts Drug Facts and Comparisons online	$ 360.00
eFacts Drug Interaction Facts online	$ 180.00
Iowa Drug Information System (CD-ROM)	$ 4,400.00
IPA (SilverPlatter)	$ 472.00
Medline (SilverPlatter) Internet only (1966+)	$21,000.00
MedTeach Software	$ 549.00
Micromedex >200 licensed bed facility	
Diseasedex	$13,200.00
Drugdex System	$15,598.00
Poisindex System	$15,477.00
Other Micromedex Databases	
CareNotes System	$10,285.00
Drug–Reax	$ 1,738.00
Kinetidex	$ 3,960.00
Martindale: The Complete Drug Reference	$ 1,848.00
PDR	$ 6,358.00
P&T Quik	$ 1,525.00
Reprorisk	$ 2,893.00

D. Major Online Vendors

Dialog
EBSCO Information Services
Gale Group
National Library of Medicine
Ovid Technologies, Inc.
OCLC First Search
SilverPlatter

*Costs are approximate and are based on 2002 figures.